GET

the

TANGO PIONEERS

A Celebration of Tango Argentino

(1910 to 1919)

David Thomas

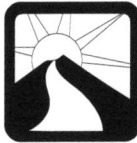

TANGO JOURNEY

David Thomas has asserted his rights to be identified as the author of this work
Copyright © 2023 by David Thomas
Editor: Marion Greenwood
Published by Tango Journey
ISBN: 978-0-9955344-3-8

Thanks and Acknowledgements

First of all to Marion who has supported, and tolerated, me in my decade-long submersion in often abstruse archive material. I am grateful for her guidance in the construction and flow of the book and for her advice that not everything that is known needs to be included.

To the Archivo General de la Nación de Argentina, the Nacional Library of Spain, and the Iberian American Institute in Berlin for their mesmerising collections of publications and photographs that have brought to life my own understanding of tango history.

To the Instituto Argentino del Tango, Buenos Aires and all of its dedicated expert lecturers and the knowledgeable fellow participants on the course *Diplomatura del Historia del Tango* (2021/22)

To the many tango researchers from across the world and across the centuries whose work has fascinated and puzzled me in equal measure.

To all in the tango scene, past and present, who have added to the magic.

And finally, to you, for choosing to get to know the Tango Pioneers. I hope that you enjoy the journey.

CONTENTS

PART ONE

The Series

Myths and the Melting Pot (Origins to 1909)
Celebration of Tango Argentino (1910 to 1919)
The Precarious Years (1920 to 1935)

Read, Listen, and Watch

Throughout this book you will see two icons: ![gramophone icon] and ![film icon] indicating that I have produced music and film clips for you on the linked YouTube Channel *Get To Know Tango*. Alongside the icon is a QR code - simply scan with your mobile phone and you will be taken directly to the film. I recommend that you read with on-line access so that you can enjoy the full multi-media experience of reading, listening, and watching[1].

Find out more on the website: *www.tango-journey.com*

---

[1] At time of publication all videos were available in all regions. It is possible that YouTube may change its policy on regional or copyright access. You should be able to locate the material via other on-line sources.

Introduction

Unfamiliar Words

If you are not from the Spanish-speaking world then there may be words used in this series that are unfamiliar to you. I have included a list with descriptions on page 212.

What is Tango?

The question is easy enough but there is no satisfactory answer. Tango is a familiar word that the general public associate with a dance, or music, and often both. Since the early 1900s there has been public discourse about the attractiveness/ugliness of tango and the descriptions of its true and distorted styles. Although we can all have our preferences none can claim to know the 'authentic' tango because quite simply such a thing has never existed. My own conclusion is that such prolonged and continuing passionate debate demonstrates that tango has always been a powerful social phenomenon that is difficult to define. Tango music and dance does exist, it is still in the melting pot, changing its ingredients, its flavours, its chefs, its consumers, and its onlookers.

There have been many attempts at formal definitions. Grove's Dictionary of Music and Musicians was first published in London in 1879. It was updated and re-published 1880, 1883, 1889, and then frequently during the first decade of the 1900s in four or five volumes. It was the most comprehensive and respected compilation of its kind and each of its lengthy and heavy volumes extended to around 800 pages. In 1910, the year of the first recording of an orquesta típica in Buenos Aires, came Grove's first entry for Tango:

A dance of Mexican origin, in which the movements of the negroes were imitated. The music is rhythmically similar in style to the Habanera, but played half as fast again, and worked up faster and faster till it ends abruptly like the conventional dances of the modern ballet. The frequent habit of writing five notes, sometimes of equal value, sometimes a dotted semiquaver, a demi-semiquaver, and a triplet of semiquavers, in the melody against four notes in the accompaniment, and vice versa, and many other varieties of rhythm of a similar nature, added to the peculiar colour of Spanish harmonical progressions which are the stamp of so-called Musica Flamenca, give it a weird fascination. The movements of the dance are less presentable to a polite audience than those of the Habanera, and as now performed in the cafés chantants of Madrid and other cities of Spain the Tango has become nothing but an incitation to desire. As such it never fails to draw forth vociferous applause. A modified form of the dance is often introduced into a Zarzuela at better-class theatres. Tangos have been written by modern composers for solo instruments, and one, by Arbos, for violin with orchestral accompaniment (also with pianoforte) is extremely graceful, refined, and characteristic.

That same definition re-appeared in each subsequent edition beyond the 1920s despite the European-wide 'tango-mania' obsession with Argentine tango that is not captured at all in the above description.

In the Argentina newspaper *Crítica* on 22 September 1913 a piece by the author (identified only as the 'Viejo Tanguero') described the origins of the dance as exotic and said that it was 'devised one day by people of colour but these days it is linked with the old traditions of vidalitas and sentimental estilos[2]'. The text is full of contradictions, chronological errors, and illogical conclusions yet extracts were frequently quoted as fact by later researchers mainly because of the confident title: *El tango, su evolución y su historia* ('The tango, its evolution and history'). The writings have been unpicked as without historic merit and certainly without evidence by respected researchers and historians Hugo Lamas and Enrique Binda with whom I find myself in agreement.

So where does this absence of an accurate definition take us? It took me to a state of resigned acceptance that any contrived definition is doomed to be inadequate. Tango (the music, the dance, the poetry, the cultural heritage) is wonderfully varied and beguilingly intangible. Over many decades the need to present a simple, understandable story of tango (what it is and where it came

---

[2] Vidalitas and estilos are folk genres

from) has produced many myths, misunderstandings, and muddles[3]: it is African, it is Italian, it is from the brothels, it was rejected by decent society, it was adopted by the upper classes following its success in Paris, and so on.

Tango does not need to be defined it just needs to be better understood. This *Get To Know* series is a presentation of facts about the origins and development of the art form that is tango and those that helped it along the way. I hope that you enjoy getting to know the tango pioneers.

---

[3] see *Get To Know the Tango Pioneers: Myths and the Melting Pot*

PART TWO

The Tango Environment

In order to understand the development of tango we must understand the pre-existing conditions from which it gradually evolved. The public was enjoying music and dance long before any identifiable notion of tango emerged and so when it did, often unnoticed, the infrastructure was already in place to allow tango to grow.

There follows two sections highlighting that fertile environment:

a) popular venues where people listened and danced to all kinds of music and where tango made its early appearances: café-bars, carnivals, theatres, and cabarets;

b) methods of broadcasting beyond the reach of those venues: recordings, sheet music, pianolas, street organs, and films.

Venues

Café-bars, carnivals, fetes, theatres, cabarets

1.   Café-bars

Café-bars, with their vast array of styles and clientele, have always been a familiar feature of everyday life in Buenos Aires. If you were to browse the fortnightly issues of the magazine *Caras y Caretas* during the years of 1910 to 1919 you would find references to café life in advertisements, fictional short stories, features, and news items. Many cafés provided their customers with musical

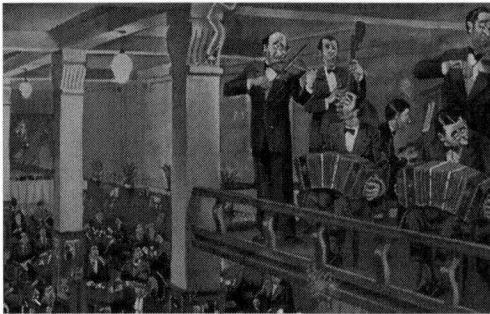

entertainment that included tango musicians and so, although some customers may not have been in the cafés in order to listen to the music, it became increasingly difficult to avoid it. From the venue's perspective all that was required was a chair for the bandoneonist and limited standing space for the violinist, flautist, and guitarist. Larger and busier venues created a performance area almost at ceiling height like a gallery (see image), that enabled all floor space below to be filled by paying customers, and increasingly through this decade, the venues that had the space found themselves investing in a piano.

The list of café-bars that are known to have hosted the tango pioneers during this decade is long and represents only a tiny sample of the true number. The myths, or misunderstandings, of tango history lead us to believe that the venues were restricted to a few of the poorer barrios particularly in the south of the city around the dock area. The evidence to the contrary is that tango was played regularly in café-bars from the city centre out to the surrounding towns and beyond to the provinces. Those cafés frequently named in connection with the pioneers include the Argentino, Atenas, Buseca, Caburé, Domínguez, Eden, Estribo, Garibotto, los Loros, Marina, Maratón, Monterrey, Morocco, Parque, and Royal. In 1914 the Café Estribo advertised itself as the only place one could hear every evening the latest creole (and foreign) music. Playing there was 'the popular and well-known pianist Roberto Firpo, the known King of the Bandoneón Eduardo Arolas, and the celebrated creole violinist Tito Roccatagliata'. The advertisement encouraged the customers to select the music that they wanted to hear simply by passing a note to the waiter, with a small payment.

Although most of the café-bars from the 1910s no longer exist the current tango tourists in Buenos Aires can apply the necessary degree of imagination to transport themselves back to those years by visiting some of the city's oldest venues, now preserved as *bares notables.*

2.   Carnivals

During the years 1905 to 1907 newspapers reported that tango music was dominating all of the carnival entertainment. There followed a two-year lull in reporting but in February 1910 the reports of tango crept back:

- although the orchestras at the Teatro Casino mainly played habaneras, vals, and an 'outstanding cake-walk' they also included a set of tangos;
- the Teatro Politeama was described in *La Nacional* as a veritable academy of tango criollo with clear variations in dance style by visitors from different barrios[4]. The watching journalist saw tango mixed with influences of the polka, the mazurka, vals, and schottische.

From 1912 to 1914 the newspapers once again started to report that tango was not only present but was taking over as the dominant carnival music. As if to celebrate its return in February 1912 *Caras y Caretas* published a whole page of colour drawings entitled 'The Triumph of Tango' that showed elegantly dressed dancing couples. In February 1914 the famous orquesta típica of Vicente Greco[5] led the carnival dance

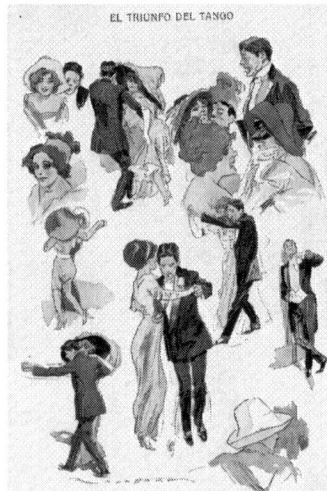

EL TRIUNFO DEL TANGO

---

[4] specific local areas of the city

[5] his group was the first to be named an 'orquesta tipíca especial criolla'

nights in the city centre Teatro Nacional Norte[6]. The musicians were Vicente himself and Juan Labissier on bandoneóns, Domingo Greco on piano, Francisco Canaro and Juan Abate on violins, and Vicente Pecci on flute. Theatres at carnival time were certainly not auditoriums with quietly attentive audiences. At a time before electric microphones and amplifiers the sextet would have struggled to have been heard in front of hundreds of revellers. Nevertheless the sextet returned in 1915 but then in 1916 they moved to the Teatro Politeama (in the city of Rosario) and more than doubled their number on stage to take acoustic control. The regular bandoneonists Vicente Greco and Juan Labissier were augmented by Pedro Polito and Osvaldo Fresedo; the violinists consisted of two Franciscos (Canaro and Confeta) and two Rafaels (Canaro and Rinaldi); the pianist was Samuel Castriota whilst another pianist José Martínez played an harmonium; the double bass was played by Leopoldo Thompson; and the woodwind section was provided by flautist Vicente Pecci and clarinetist Juan Carlos Bazán. Also on stage was Pablo Laise who provided what was known as the 'lija' - a percussive scratching sound. Francisco Canaro later said that it was at that carnival that the tango orquesta típica became culturally acceptable in Rosario, leading thereafter to him being invited to play at venues such as the Savoy Hotel in Rosario.

The following year, 1917, the organisers of the carnival in Rosario wanted to fill their prestigious Teatro Colón with revellers and needed an extra-large orchestra to produce the necessary volume. In order to satisfy the public demand it had to be a tango orchestra. There was no such orchestra in existence and so they travelled to Buenos Aires and met, in the Cabaret Montmartre, the leaders of

---

[6] where today stands the magnificent bookshop El Ateneo Grand Splendid

two quintets: Roberto Firpo and Francisco Canaro. The organisers made an attractive business proposal that convinced the two bandleaders to merge their quintets and to find additional musicians in order to form the grand Orquesta Típica Criolla Firpo-Canaro. The posters advertising the event showed photographs of the main musicians[7] and promised a selection of 200 tangos, which was at least ten hours of performances. The names of the musicians on that stage was a staggering collection of the best and the music that must have powered out leaves me yearning for the miracle of time travel. That would be the year, the place, and the moment for me. On the stage were pianists Roberto Firpo and José Martínez, the bandoneón line-up was Eduardo Arolas, Osvaldo Fresedo, Juan Deambroggio, Minotto Di Cicco, and Pedro Polito; the violinists were Francisco Canaro, Julio Doutry, Agesilao Ferrazzano, and Cayetano Puglisi; Leopoldo Thompson provided the double bass; with flautist Alejandro Michetti and Juan Carlos Bazán on clarinet. Every musician on that stage was a tango maestro that shaped the sound and the soul of the tango music that went on to keep people dancing at milongas around the world for more than a century.

3.   Fetes

A romería (originally a pilgrimiage to honour a saint) was a public festival with a vast array of entertainment, food, drink, dance, and song. It is no surprise that where ordinary people gathered there was also tango. On 14 September 1912 *Caras y Caretas* published images from the recent romería:

---

[7] some accounts say that although Tito Roccatagliata was advertised he did not appear and had been replaced by the 15 year old Cayetano Puglisi

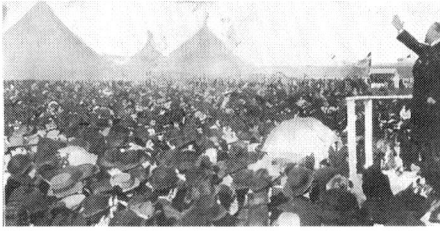

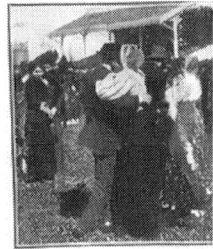

Bailando un tango.

4.   Theatres

The audiences of the city theatres were large in number and came from a wide and varied section of society. They may not all have been early adopters of tango music and dance but they were nevertheless exposed to it and entertained by it.

The playwright and producer Carlos Pacheco had first caused a sensation in 1906 with his sympathetic portrayal of conventillo life, compadritos, anarchists, and the tango dance. In 1910 (at a time of street protests, strikes, and anarchist violence) his play *De Hombre a Hombre* tried to shift society's perception of poor people from being lazy and criminal to them being valued as honest and hard working. The by-product of his efforts was the wider social acceptance of musicians from the poorer barrios. His productions were so successful, and the songs from his shows so popular, that he spent two busy days in March 1910 singing them to the accompaniment of a guitar in a makeshift studio with visiting Victor recording engineer Raymond Sooy. He recorded at least 30 tracks that included a range of creole genres: vidalitas, tristes, estilos, marches, some comic narrations, milongas and a tango. Despite the paucity of tangos in his recordings the *Caras y Caretas* magazine in August

1910 informed its readers that of all of the variants of creole music in the theatre productions it was tango that was the musical 'piece de resistance'. The article named the enduring tangos *Bartolo* and *La morocha* and added that even in the more highly cultured productions in the theatres of La Scala and the Royal there was always some visiting French singer adopting a porteño nasal tone to deliver the obligatory tango.

Pacheco continued to produce similarly themed plays in the heart of the Buenos Aires theatre land. His 1912 play *Pajaras de Presa* told the tale of a young woman from the conventillos who improved her prospects by becoming a 'milonguera' in a rather modest café, singing and dancing tango, and being a hostess to the male customers. Within the play were other social observations about the role of the rich boys (the so-called 'niños bien') mixing with the conventillo girls, the cynical anarchists, and the uneducated Italian immigrants with their comical distortions of Spanish (called 'cocoliche' after a real actor who spoke in such a way). The play did not disapprove of the milongueras' lifestyle but used it as an example of the limited opportunities for working class women to improve their living conditions and life opportunities. Any implied or explicit reference to the milongueras' link to prostitution was not a damning critique of their morals but an indictment of the social injustices leading to their plight. That same theme continued through the following years, for example in his 1917 play *Barracas* the female protagonist left her life in the barrio with few prospects and became a milonguera. The same theme can still be found in the lyrics of tangos that are heard and danced in today's milongas - such as *Milonguita* and *Margot:*

- 'You were born in the misery of the arrabal conventillo....now between the cigar smoke and the champagne of the Armenonville ....you are no longer my Margarita, now they call you Margot' *Margot* (1919);

• 'And between the wine and the last tango a rich guy takes you back to his apartment, how alone you feel and when you cry they say it is because of the champagne' *Milonguita* (1920).

The original reason for using the imagery of prostitution in order to highlight social injustice was eventually forgotten and became one of the main misleading clichés and imagery of tango.

Following the lead of Carlos Pacheco, Alberto Vacarezza soon became an influential playwright whose themes were also mainly set in and around the conventillos. According to his own descriptions his plays always featured Italian immigrants, innocent girls, compadritos, flirts, jealousy, fights, stabbings, shootings, and the police. As a result of his vice-ridden themes some in the middle class audiences came

Alberto B. Vacarezza

away from the plays with a negative view of the working class musicians and their style of tango. Nevertheless Vacarezza was a promoter of tango and on 24 November 1911 at the Teatro Nacional he opened his play *Los Escrushantes* that included characters dancing tango with 'cortes'[8]. The leading lady was Olinda Bozán, who later sang and recorded a few tangos with the orchestra of Francisco Canaro in 1928/9[9].

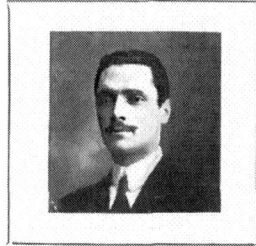

---

[8] sharp movements that became associated with street tango although were moves borrowed from other popular dances.

[9] Olinda and her younger cousin Sofía became popular tango singers on stage and in film from the 1920s to 1950s

Alberto Vacarezza not only produced plays but also wrote the lyrics of tangos appearing in them. He was later celebrated and photographed in an article entitled 'The Tango Poets' (*Caras y Caretas* 8 May 1926) in which he was described as a famous man of the theatre who had obtained magnificent success with the lyrics of his tangos such as:

- *La Copa del Olvido* recorded much later by Ricardo Tanturi (1942) and by Rodolfo Biagi (1952); and
- *No Le Digas Que La Quiero* recorded by Biagi (1940), Aníbal Troilo (1941), and Alfredo De Angelis (1955).

Despite the valiant attempts by many playwrights to make satirical political commentary the audiences appeared to be there simply to enjoy the tangos. It was becoming more difficult to find plays, regardless of their subject matter, that did not include tangos. In December 1916 the magazine *La Razón* reviewed the opening of the play *La Cena de los Gaviones* (by Roberto Cayol) and observed that the satire and cynical humour passed by unnoticed but not so the tangos, one of which was played on a harmonium. Another review that month (in *La Epoca*) noted that the entire audience from the most expensive to the cheapest seats demanded three times the repeated performance of the 'tango arrabalero' danced to a milonga played on guitar. Such audience enthusiasm continued to be reported for years to come, for example, in the review of the 1922 play *El Bailarin de Cabaret* the singer Ignacio Corsini had to repeat one of his tangos an unsettling five times.

In 1918 the play, *Cuidado con los ladrones* (Beware of the thieves) by Alberto Novión, included musicians playing tango at a party in the conventillo with the usual characters present (compadritos, thieves, and anarchists). That same year a softer perspective was introduced in the play *Los Dientes del Perro* when one character sang *Mi Noche*

Triste that was later classified (by some) as the first 'tango cancion'[10]. The play was co-written by José González Castillo (left) and Alberto Weisbach (centre) and produced by Elías Alippi (right). The original stage directions read 'Curtain rises. Interior of a cabaret, the orquesta típica is on a wooden platform. Chairs, tables and everything else is in the usual layout. Scene One the cabaret is in full swing.' It opened on 26 April 1918 at the Teatro Nacional and the magazine *La Mañana* reported how the presence of the orchestra on the stage as part of the cabaret scene (as opposed to being in the orchestra pit) gave a novel and interesting spin to the play.

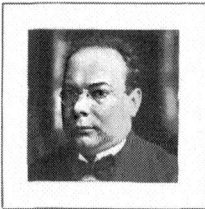

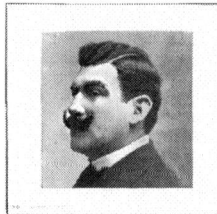

José Gonzáles Castillo   Alberto F. Weisbach   ELIAS ALIPPI

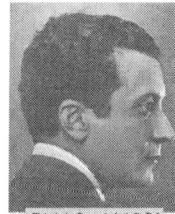

Our interest in that development is heightened because the orchestra was led by the pioneer tango pianist Roberto Firpo. The magazine *El Hogar* reported the liveliness of the orchestra with its playful use of unusual sound effects such as a car horn and calls of encouragement from the musicians to the dancers. Occasionally at today's milongas the dancers will also hear recordings of tango musicians calling out and making some quite comical noises particularly in the recordings from the late 1920s by the orchestras of Roberto Firpo, Julio De Caro, and the Orquestas Típicas

---

[10] See *Part Four Pioneers/Lyricists*

Brunswick and Victor. The review in *El Hogar* went on to note that one musician was playing the 'acordeón or mandoneón as it is called'. The word 'bandoneón' took several more years to settle in to accepted use. You can watch below a representation of that April 1918 scene in the 1949 film *La Historia del Tango*. Although the 1949 film version is more staid than the original stage performance the pianist is at least Roberto Firpo himself, then 65 years old.

The innovation of placing a tango orchestra on the stage caught on quickly and others followed, such as in *La Boca del Riachuelo* and *El Cabaret Montmartre*. The latter opened at the Teatro Nacional from 25 June to 1 September 1919 and the orchestra members were Roberto Firpo (piano), Cayetano Puglisi (violin), Pedro Maffia and Juan Bautista Deambroggio (bandoneóns), and a drummer. The play continued beyond September 1919 but the original musicians moved on to other commitments and were replaced by Ángel D'Agostino (piano), Juan D'Arienzo and Alfredo Mazzeo (violins), and two bandoneonists - the experienced José Arturo Severino and Nicolás Primiani.

Other plays up to 1919 not only featured tango life in the storyline but often had 'tango' in their titles to be sure to draw in the crowds:
- *El Alma del Tango* (1914) by Roberto Lino Cayol who had first established himself as a leading playwright in 1909 and became a leading tango lyricist. Roberto was the son of Carlos Cayol, co-owner of the telephone and telegraph company Cayol & Newman who were the first to

manufacture the Edison Talking Machines in Argentina (in 1878);

- *El Tango en Buenos Aires* (1914) by Enrique García Velloso;
- *El Cabaret* (1914) by Carlos Pacheco;
- *El Patio de Las Flores* (1915) by Armando Discépolo;
- *La Pebeta del Bar Copetín* (1917) by José González Castillo;
- *Tangos, Tongos y Tungos* (1918) by Carlos Pacheco;
- *El Tango en París* (1918) by Enrique García Velloso.

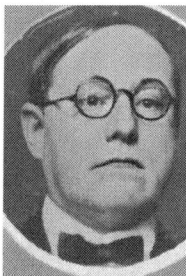

E G Velloso

5.   Cabarets

The concept of cabarets arrived in Buenos Aires from trend-setting Paris. On 22 November 1913 the magazine *Caras y Caretas* published an article on 'The invasion of the cabaret' in to Buenos Aires nightlife making fun of the pretentious Parisian airs of the owners, staff, and clientele. It mocked the men for dressing in tuxedos, the ladies for their elegant gowns, the drinking of champagne as being *de rigueur*, and the dancing of tango in the Parisian style. The provision of cabaret music had changed from being just a solo pianist, to a resident band, and then to the tango specialism of the orquesta típica. The tango musicians, regardless of their working-class status, had to dress appropriately in dinner jackets or tuxedos. From at least 1913 there are photographs of tango musicians wearing bow ties as if to assure their respectable credentials but closer inspection often reveals poorer quality, creased lounge suits. In June 1919 at the Teatro Nacional the play *El Cabaret Montmartre* showed the mockingly comic scene of tango musicians dressed in hired dinner jackets but knowing neither how to wear them nor how to behave in an elegant situation. Towards the 1930s it became usual to see tango musicians wearing dinner jackets as, in order to work, they needed to conform to the expectations of the moneyed class. As late as 1951 Enrique Santos Discépolo criticised the upper-classes for dressing up street tango musicians in tuxedos and hijacking the music of the poor whilst not having any interest in their lives nor their welfare. And so it had been since at least 1910.

There was no shortage of cabarets providing venues for tango bands during this period and a few have remained particularly prominent in the history of tango:

- the Armenonville opened in late 1911 in the barrio of lower Palermo/upper Recoleta. It was described at the time as a cabaret and a restaurant with the finest artists and finest foods for the city's finest people. It was built in the style of a colonial chalet set in gardens with a large outside space for dining and inside was an elegant dance salon with chandeliers and full-length mirrors. If we were to believe the myth of the rejection of tango by the Argentinian upper-classes then we would be surprised to hear that shortly after its opening the Armenonvillle owners invited the tango band of Vicente Greco to perform. Juan Maglio also performed there in 1912.

Furthermore, he composed and recorded his tribute 'Tango brillante' entitled *Armenonville* (with the cover of the sheet music illustrating the grand roadside entrance to the building). In 1913 the Armenonville auditioned and recruited its own house tango quartet led by Roberto Firpo who played there his tango compositions *Alma de bohemio, Sentimiento criollo, De pura cepa* and others that are still well known today;

- the Tabarín entertained its patrons with tango bands that included the trio of Roberto Firpo with bandoneonist Eduardo Arolas and violinist Tito Roccatagliatta;

- the Abbaye had the bandoneonist Augusto Berto playing with flautist Luis Teisseire and violinist Pelegrino Paulos and in 1918 the resident pianist was the refined Juan Carlos Cobían;

- the Cabaret Maxim had the pianist Pascual Cardarópoli in a tango trio. Cardarópoli composed the tango *La Sonámbula* that has its place in tango history as the first bandoneón solo recording (see the section on Juan Maglio below);

- the customers at the Montmartre cabaret in 1916 were entertained by the Francisco Canaro band. It was there that Leopoldo Thompson enlivened the performances by striking the strings of his double bass with the bow and the instrument's wooden body with the flat of his hand (just as he had done years before with his guitar), calling out enthusiastically to energise both the band and the guests.

Broadcasting

Recordings, sheet music, pianolas, organitos, films

1. Recordings

The global leaders in the recording and manufacture of discs and the production of talking machines were based in North America, Germany, and England. Their engineers toured the world with portable recording equipment to capture local artists, then sent the masters back home where their factories manufactured bulk quantities of discs labelled in the language of the destination country. There were few places in the world that the visiting teams did not reach. In Argentina, like everywhere else, there were leading entrepreneurs who became the in-country agents and distributors. They provided the local artists; the premises for the visiting engineers to convert to a recording laboratory; and stocked, promoted, and sold the end-product records and talking machines. The main Buenos Aires entrepreneurs during this period were: Juan and José Tagini (Columbia), Alfredo Améndola (Atlanta), Max Glücksmann (Odeon), Carlos Nasca (ERA), and the retailer J.J. Pratt (Victor).

The first tango discs had been recorded in Buenos Aires in 1902 and the first recorded orquesta típica with a bandoneón in 1909[11]. The years to 1914 saw increased investment and trade between the Buenos Aires agents and European, mainly German, record

---

[11] See Part Four below: *Bandoneonists/Greco*

companies but those relying on the cross-Atlantic trade at the start of the World War (1914-1918) saw all of their previous arrangements come to halt. They had to find alternative arrangements and initially their saviours were similar entrepreneurs in Brazil (Fred Figner and Saverio Leonetti) who were ahead of the game and had already established their own recording and disc manufacturing facilities.

Music recordings around the world were all made in more or less the same way. The musicians assembled around one large horn in to which flowed their combined sound. The resulting vibrations were captured and transferred to a stylus that etched a groove in to a rotating wax master cylinder or disc. Any mixing or balancing of instruments could only be done beforehand by adjusting the positions of each musician in relation to the listening horn. Prior to recording, the sound technician could pre-listen by using earpieces attached by a rubber tube at the base of the horn. He could then make changes to the physical positions of the musicians and/or adding or removing particular instruments. The musicians were not only arranged by distance from the horn and from each other but also by elevation. Platforms were built for some, high stools for others. In the Buenos Aires magazine *Caras y Caretas* on 24 July 1909 an article described the recording process and how the piano in particular needed to be carefully placed, usually on a platform. For many years the attempted inclusion of the piano with other instruments created such an overwhelming sound distortion that in early recordings of the tango orquestas típicas the piano was often replaced by a guitar. In that way the recordings did not accurately reflect the sound of the group's live performances. Additionally the recording process could only deal with a limited range of audio frequencies and so the artists were instructed to choose a repertoire within that range or to alter the way they normally played their regular music. Many techniques were tried to improve the recording capabilities such as varying the recording horns by shape, size, material, and location. The technicians discovered that wooden horns were best for guitars and other stringed instruments whilst bronze was better for the clarity of voices and brass bands. Cardboard horns were also introduced in an attempt to soften the metallic sound on the disc. Other experimental variations concerned the needle types, the rotation speeds, and the wax thickness. Recording rooms had to be hot to keep the wax soft enough to receive the minuscule vibrations of the needle yet it could not be too hot otherwise the wax would not maintain its shape. There was not the technological capability to set and maintain a perfect temperature and so uncontrolled variations also affected the resulting sound transfer.

When making judgements about the quality of the music produced by the tango pioneers the modern listener should take in to account all of the technical restrictions in the recording laboratory (just a standard room crudely adapted with curtains to muffle outside noise) as well as the subsequent deterioration due to the recordings' age, careless storage, and degree of accurate reproduction over the following decades when transferring to media such as vinyl, tape, compact disc, and digital. We will never be able to hear the pioneers as they sounded when they played in the bars and cafés of Buenos Aires but we can imagine them and be sure that they would have gripped us immediately.

When the records were released there was an eager and excited public waiting for them. The availability, affordability, and popularity of recordings had been increasing year on year to such an extent that between 1908 and 1913 it is estimated that in homes, cafés, dance halls, theatres, and a wide range of retail and other businesses across Argentina there were nearly 200,000 gramophones and about 10 million discs and cylinders. It is estimated that in 1910 alone nearly 2 million tango records were purchased.

Tagini & Columbia

On 15 November 1909 the North American trade magazine *Talking Machine World* reported that William Freiburg and his assistant Gus Forbush of Columbia Phonograph's laboratory recording staff, had set sail from New York for Buenos Aires to make vocal and instrumental records. They based themselves at the Casa Tagini, 924 Avenida de Mayo, Buenos Aires and once their mission was completed and had returned to the USA in April 1910, Ed Burns (the manager of the Columbia Export Department in the USA) said that the Buenos Aires recordings from Freiburg and Forbush were 'the finest and very best records made in that part of the world'. Amongst the tangos they recorded by different artists were those of particular historic significance: in July 1910 Casa Tagini placed the first advertisement for the first record released by the first Orquesta Típica Criolla Especial, being the first to include a bandoneón[12].

In early 1912 Tagini and Columbia established a permanent recording facility in Buenos Aires putting them in a leading position amongst competitors who had to either rely on the occasional visiting recording engineer with portable (inferior) equipment or to send their artists abroad to record. The new Tagini recording laboratory was revealed to the public in an article on 17 May 1912, together with photographs showing it in action. A

---

[s] see below Bandoneonists/Greco.

pianist was on an elevated platform, a singer facing directly in to the listening horn, whilst beside him stood a violinist (with attached cornet for amplification). In another photograph a band of some 20 musicians were squeezed in to the room at different elevations in front of the single recording horn. One photograph in particular reveals the extent of sound experimentation. The singing guitarists

Saúl Salinas (who would soon become a mentor to the young Carlos Gardel) and Auguste de Giuli stood in front of not one but at least four recording horns: two pointing down to their guitars and two up to their mouths. It is likely that the material of the horns were different (metal for the voices and wood or even cardboard for the guitars). Standing-by in the corner were other horns of different sizes,

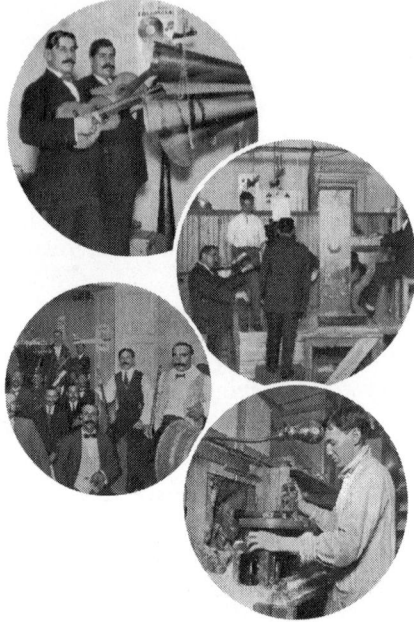

materials, and designs in case that combination did not produce the required tonality and balance. All of the listening horns narrowed to a single place behind a wooden panel where the combined sound merged to a single diaphragm that agitated the single needle that etched its vibrations in to the warm rotating wax. The creation of the master disc was watched over by a specialist engineer wearing a long white laboratory coat. In November 1912 *Talking*

Machine World said that José Tagini was 'considered to be the largest dealer in the world'. That is an astounding claim for this one retail business in Buenos Aires. The article said that its stock of records in its prestigious store and in its multi-storey warehouse, amounted to half a million. In 1912/1913 Columbia, from its Buenos Aires headquarters in Casa Tagini, were distributing not only to most (if not all) South and Central American countries but also to Spain. Nevertheless the Tagini/Columbia partnership did not have the capability to manufacture the discs and still relied on its arrangements with Germany. At the pinnacle of Tagini's fortunes disaster struck with the commencement of the First World War from which Tagini never recovered and disappeared from the story of the recording pioneers.

Améndola & Atlanta

Alfredo Améndola, born in Italy and raised in Buenos Aires, was a musician with an entrepreneurial spirit and (like everybody else) had no idea of the looming geo-political crisis in Europe. In 1912 he sailed across the Atlantic to Germany and negotiated with the International Talking Machine company that traded as Odeon. He returned with the necessary licence, equipment to record masters, an engineer to help him, and a contract to send the masters back to Germany for the production of his records. The discs were to be double-sided and the labels pre-printed in Spanish ready for the Argentinian market. On Monday 31 March 1913 Améndola opened his first retail premises in the front of the (former) Teatro San Martín at 274 Esmeralda. On 5 April he placed his first advertisement launching his new Atlanta label. His entry in to the market was neither gentle nor subtle. Half of his full page advertisement was an extraordinary attack on the general offerings of others, namely 'the unscrupulous foreign companies that only fill their own pockets at the expense of the public and sell cheap and poor quality records of purportedly national artists'. He promised that his company, Atlanta, would make every sacrifice to ensure that Argentina did not remain a market for the 'bad and the cheap' by offering the true and pure spirit of the Pampas to those households with good taste. He declared that the public would be convinced, with well-founded pride, that no longer did they need to look abroad for plentiful good quality music and that Atlanta was a patriotic work that cemented the national spirit.

I get the strong feeling that, apart from the German technician, Améndola was working alone as surely a second opinion may have toned down the uninhibited attack on his fellow record distributors. He did have an opportunity to think again when he published another full-page advertisement the following week. He decided to be consistent: 'some of our competitors having realised the indisputable superiority of Atlanta records have tried to undermine them but all in vain…the respectable intelligent public have heard the discs and remain convinced of their unbeatable quality'. He invited the readers to come and listen for free, without any obligation to buy, to the recordings of the 'Quintetos Criollos' of Augusto (Berto), Garrote (Greco), Firpo, Bevilacqua, Tano Genaro (Espósito) and both the Rondalla Atlanta and the Banda Atlanta (directed by Arturo Bassi). The quintets were described as such because when they performed live there were five musicians but the discs were only quartets or trios because the recording capabilities required them to drop the piano and/or the flute, and adopt whatever instrument grouping the recording engineer thought best.

It appears that June was the month that Améndola employed an enthusiastic marketing adviser who from the following week and for the rest of the year produced particularly innovative, eye-catching and frankly unique advertisements compared to all the other record retailers. The compilation shown (below) was published on 3 January 1914.

In August and September 1913 his advertisements included the 'most famous 'rondallas criollas'[13] led by Augusto (Berto), Garrote (Vicente Greco), Tano Genaro (Espósito); and 'the famous Firpo'. Sadly only a few of the tangos listed are known to us today but we must not conclude that they were not good enough to survive the following decades but simply that our exposure to the most popular tango music of that time is frustratingly limited. On 27 September 1913 Améndola declared 'Just arrived are the famous compositions of Firpo played on Bandoleón, violins etc and directed by the famous author himself'. The misspelling of the bandoneón during the first 15 years of the century is not uncommon as both the name and the sound were still largely unfamiliar. It was not until 22 November 1913 that Améndola first mentioned the descriptive term 'orquesta típicas criollas' in which he offered the tangos of Vicente Greco, Genaro Espósito, and

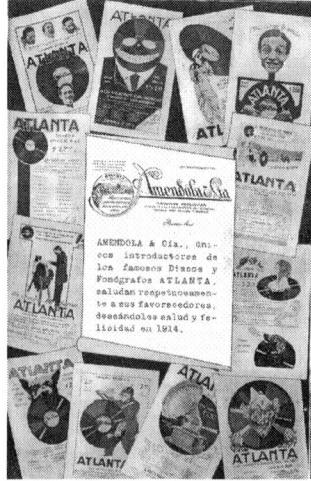

---

[13] they were not rondallas (groups of stringed instruments) but orquestas típicas with bandoneón. Terminology was neither consistent nor accurate.

Augusto Berto. Those titles still known to modern day tango fans were *El entrerriano*, *Rodríguez Peña*, and *Sentimiento criollo*. On 4 October Améndola's promotion of the tango *Sentimiento criollo* by Roberto Firpo (right) is shown to be fascinating a group of well-dressed children who have abandoned their toys to stare excitedly at the sound coming from the horn. Not only was Améndola offering tangos by Firpo, Espósito, Berto and others to middle-class homes who could afford gramophones but such was the social acceptance of tango from the arrabal[14] played on the 'bandoleón' that he used the entertainment of young children as a marketing tool. This is an image that undermines the myth that such tangos were shunned from decent homes.

Business for Améndola was slowing down and shipments from Germany could not be guaranteed due to the inevitable wartime disruptions. The losses and risks to shipping had become too great to maintain the business model of sending masters and records back and forth across the Atlantic. His resulting financial difficulties ultimately meant that in 1916 he had to sell his stock and recording equipment. The opportunist buyer was Max Glücksmann, about whom we shall read more shortly. Despite the

---

[14] lower-class areas, see Unfamiliar Words p212

collapse of his business Améndola did continue to trade beyond that date using recording facilities in Porto Alegre, Brazil (see below) but despite finding an alternative manufacturer, signing up many of the top tango musicians, and recording many of the best compositions Alfredo Améndola's Atlanta business finally ceased to trade in 1917[15].

Glücksmann & Odeon
Prior to 1914 Max Glücksmann of the retailer Casa Lepage had been an agent for Victor gramophones and records. Suddenly on 28 March 1914, the very next publication of *Caras y Caretas* after Améndola's last advertisement, Glücksmann placed a double-page advertisement for 'the most notable creole records that exist'. He was now not just a retail agent but, having obtained the equipment and contacts from Améndola, he was recording local musicians at his premises on the Avenida Callao in central Buenos Aires. He claimed to be sending the master discs to the International Talking Machine Company in North America but I suspect that they went instead to the record factory in Brazil for production on the Odeon label[16].

Glücksmann emphasised his guarantee that Odeon records were neither pirated copies nor those fraudulently masquerading as famous musicians. He printed signed letters by the artists, together with their photographs, praising Odeon's quality recording process and its efforts to prove authenticity. The advertisement assured readers that 'the creole records of Odeon are signed by the

---

[15] he then set up the Casa Electra and the Tele-phone label
[16] Over the coming decades Glücksmann changed the branding from Odeon, to Nacional Odeon, and then to Nacional. The changing nomenclature was not consistent and so where you see any of the variations be assured that it refers to the same Glüksmann enterprise.

maestros who direct the musicians giving them a stamp of guarantee and special exclusivity plus in some cases, like those of Arolas and Firpo, they are also composers of the works. Any record without their signatures is not authentic'. Glücksmann was not the first to engrave the artist's signature on the master discs and to warn against imitation. In October 1898 a USA Zon-o-phone advertisement declared that the embossed signature of its artists was a guarantee of authenticity and further warned against the manufacture, resale or purchase of unscrupulous imitations threatening all with prosecution (including the buying customer). The world of light entertainment was clearly delivered by some heavy-handed business practices. There is evidence of recordings having been copied without authority and re-sold on different labels (pirated) and recordings of unknown musicians being mis-described as reputable artists. Glücksmann's marketing campaign, ostensibly to protect the public from poor quality products, successfully established his public image as a reliable and well-connected music promoter whilst at the same time undermined trust in his competitors.

In 1914 Glücksmann also recorded other, today lesser known, names:

- the Orquesta Típica Rodríguez. Alberto Rodríguez became second bandoneonist with Osvaldo Fresedo on his 1927/1928 recordings. The violinist was José Pecora who composed many tangos only a few of which we know today, for example *Amando en silencio*, recorded by Edgardo Donato (1941);
- the Orquesta Típica Criolla Pécora that was probably the same musicians as that of Rodríguez but the change of name filled the catalogue with ostensibly more artists;
- the Orquesta Típica Criolla Roccatagliata which was probably the same as the Firpo quartet;
- the Orquesta Típica El Rusito directed by Antonio Guzman on bandoneón, with Rafael Tuegols (violin), Luis Aluisin (flute) and Roque Ardit (guitar); and
- the Orquesta Típica Criolla Union, sometimes referred to as the Cuarteto Union, directed by bandoneonist Leopoldo Ruíz, with Julian Urdapilleta (violin), José Guerriero (flute) and Luciano Ríos (guitar).

There was no shortage in Buenos Aires of competent tango musicians however from 1915 to 1919 in every *Caras y Caretas* publication Glücksmann's Casa Lepage advertisements featured Roberto Firpo as the main, often only, tango recording artist. It is worth pausing to consider the supremely dominant commercial status that Firpo enjoyed amongst his peers and in the eyes of the record buying public (for whom tango equalled Roberto Firpo).

Glücksmann's business was not only based in Buenos Aires. In 1916 he placed an advertisement in the Uruguay magazine *Pagina Blanca* for his music shop 'Casa Lepage de Max Glücksmann' based in the city centre of Montevideo. Unsurprisingly on sale were double-sided discs on the Odeon label recorded of course by the Orquesta Típica Criolla Roberto Firpo that included Firpo's own compositions *El amanecer, Didi, El apronte, El horizonte*.

During the World War years (1914 to 1918) Glücksmann had arranged with the Germany-based Odeon to send his recordings to their recently opened Brazilian factory for the manufacture of the discs [17]. The arrangement not only allowed Glücksmann to continue growing his business but he also quickly realised the potential benefits of having his own record factory in Buenos Aires. In 1919 construction work began on an Odeon factory (in San Fernando just 15 kilometres to the north of the Buenos Aires city centre) under Glücksmann's control with the full range of equipment to record and to manufacture discs. Glücksmann started to sign local musicians and composers to long term exclusive contracts, thereby restricting access by his competitors, particularly the North American Victor Talking Machine Company [18]. Furthermore he started to control a large part of the sales of sheet music, built an empire of cinemas where his contracted tango musicians provided the sound to silent films, and in 1924 he became a pioneer of the tango radio scene.

---

[17] see below *World War 1 and Brazil*

[18] Odeon's foothold in Buenos Aires was challenged by a new production factory built in 1924 by the USA Victor company.

Victor

In 1910 the Victor Talking Machine Company made their second recording expedition to Argentina[19] by sending Raymond Sooy, an expert engineer (but a disappointing diarist). On 30 January 1910 Sooy sailed from New York on the ship *SS Verdi*, arrived in Buenos Aires on 14 February, stayed for three months, made 424 recordings and returned home on the *SS Vasari*. His diary presents us with detail concerning the fun he had on board the ships but absolutely no details of the artists nor of the recording sessions. We do not know for certain where in Buenos Aires he made his recordings but do know that in 1910 the main retailers of Victor products were Casa Tagini and Casa Lepage (Glücksmann). We also know that from 25 February to 6 April 1910 his recordings included the tangos: *El incendio* by the Banda del Pabellón de las Rosas; *El esquinazo, El otario* and *Hotel Victoria* by the Estudiantina Centenario; *Mi china* and *Rico tipo* by the Banda del 6 Regimiento de Infantería; *La morocha* by Dolores Candales; *Bolada de aficionado, La catrera* and several others by the Orquesta de la Sociedad Orquestal; and many non-tangos by Ángel Villoldo, Arturo de Nava, José Razzano, Linda Thelma, Eugenio Lopez, and others.

In January until March 1912 the Victor recording engineers Henry Hagen and his 18-year-old assistant Charles Althouse were in Buenos Aires. The recorded artists included Diego Munilla, Arturo and Juan Navas, Ignacio Corsini, the Banda de la Pabellón de las Rosas, and the orquesta típica Genaro Espósito. A tiny percentage of the 500 recordings were tangos.

---

[19] The first was in 1907

In January 1914 the retailer J.J. Pratt first advertised the Victrola gramophone and was the 'only and exclusive distributor in Argentina' of records and machines from the Victor Talking Machine Company. By that time the previous agent Casa Tagini was primarily engaged with Columbia and Casa Lepage (Glücksmann) with Odeon. The retailer Dellzoppa & Morixe in Montevideo was appointed by Victor as their sole agent in Uruguay and all advertisements for Victor products from 1915 through to the 1920s were issued in the joint names of Pratt, Dellzoppa & Morixe. Being outlets of North American products the initial offerings of dance music were mainly Turkey Trots, Fox Trots, Two Steps, One Step, Hesitation, Maxixe, and only some Tangos. On 6 November 1915 they advertised their first tango records by the Argentinian orquestas típicas (with 'bandoleón') of Vicente Loduca and Genaro Espósito. These were not new recordings as Loduca had been recorded in the USA in 1914 and Espósito in Buenos Aires in 1912. The years passed without any further Victor recordings in Buenos Aires and so the Argentinian music continued to be provided by the orquesta típica based in New Jersey, headed by pianist Celestino Ferrer. In order to highlight the music's local connection the Pratt, Dellzoppa & Morixe adverts gave prominence to the composers who at least did live and work in Buenos Aires/Montevideo. The advert (above) appeared on 12 February 1916 showing two portrait photographs of composers Roberto Firpo and F.J. Lomuto, being the main attraction rather than the orchestra in (much) smaller print.

After a long negotiation Victor agreed to send engineers to install recording equipment in the Pratt premises (205-217 Calle San Martin) [20] and to make recordings of local artists. On 3 March 1917 the engineers George Cheney & Charles Althouse sailed on the ship *SS Tennyson* from New York to Buenos Aires and in April and May recorded about 200 tracks including the orquestas típicas of Eduardo Arolas, Juan Maglio, Vicente Loduca (with musicians Francisco Canaro and Osvaldo Fresedo), Augusto Berto, José Severino, Alonso-Minotto, and the pianist Enrique Delfino[21]. Pratt, Dellzoppa & Morixe jointly placed a double-page advertisement on 8 December 1917 announcing 'New Victor Discs recorded in Argentina'. The first page (below) had four segments with the heading 'The most famous composers and directors of creole music orchestras'. The photographed artists were Juan Maglio, Augusto Berto, Francisco Canaro, and Eduardo Arolas who (in individually signed letters) all expressed their immense satisfaction at the quality, sharpness and exact reproduction of the recordings. The master of self-promotion Francisco Canaro additionally found space in his brief letter to mention that he was also the director of the Loduca orchestra's recordings.

---

[20] Dellazoppa & Morixe was a distribution agent in Montevideo but the only recording facilities were in the Pratt premises in Buenos Aires.
[21] see *Part Four/Pioneers* below

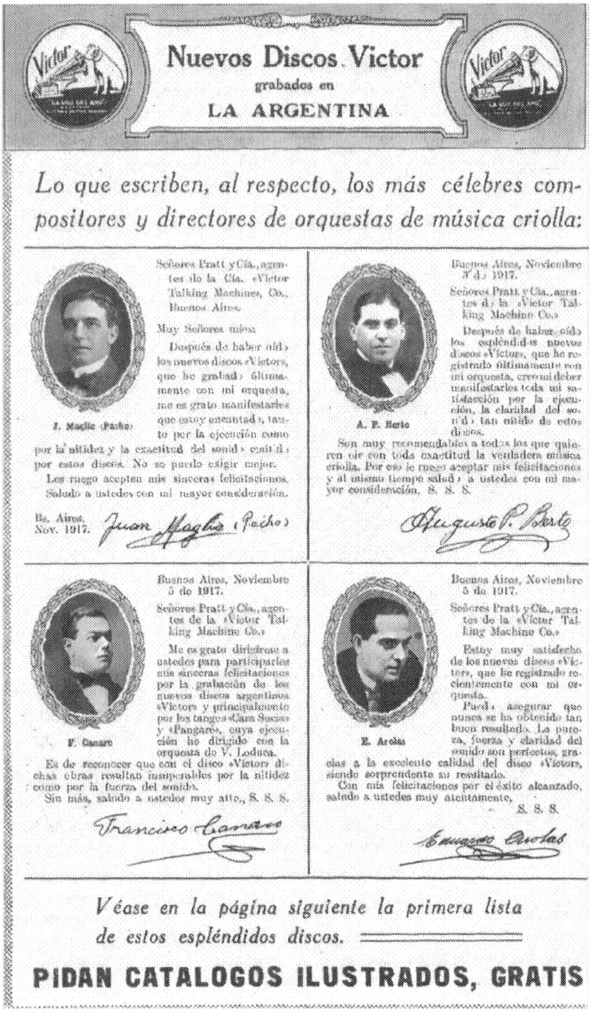
Victor
Nuevos Discos Victor
grabados en
LA ARGENTINA
Victor
Lo que escriben, al respecto, los más célebres compositores y directores de orquestas de música criolla:
Señores Pratt y Cía., agentes de la Cía. «Victor Talking Machines, Co., Buenos Aires.
Muy Señores míos:
Después de haber oído los nuevos discos «Victor», que he grabado últimamente con mi orquesta, me es grato manifestarles que estoy encantado, tanto por la ejecución como por la nitidez y la exactitud del sonido emitido por estos discos. No se puede exigir mejor.
Les ruego acepten mis sinceras felicitaciones.
Saludo a ustedes con mi mayor consideración.
J. Maglio (Pacho)
Bs. Aires, Nov. 1917.
Juan Maglio (Pacho)
Buenos Aires, Noviembre 3 de 1917.
Señores Pratt y Cía., agentes de la «Victor Talking Machine Co.»
Después de haber oído los espléndidos nuevos discos «Victor», que he registrado últimamente con mi orquesta, creo mi deber manifestarles toda mi satisfacción por la ejecución, la claridad del sonido tan nítido de estos discos.
Son muy recomendables a todos los que quieren oír con toda exactitud la verdadera música criolla. Por eso le ruego aceptar mis felicitaciones y al mismo tiempo saludo a ustedes con mi mayor consideración. S. S. S.
A. P. Berto
Augusto P. Berto
Buenos Aires, Noviembre 5 de 1917.
Señores Pratt y Cía., agentes de la «Victor Talking Machine Co.»
Me es grato dirigirme a ustedes para participarles mis sinceras felicitaciones por la grabación de los nuevos discos argentinos «Victor» y principalmente por los tangos «Cara Sucia» y «Pangaré», cuya ejecución he dirigido con la orquesta de V. Loduca.
Es de reconocer que con el disco «Victor» dichas obras resultan insuperables por la nitidez como por la fuerza del sonido.
Sin más, saludo a ustedes muy atto., S. S. S.
F. Canaro
Francisco Canaro
Buenos Aires, Noviembre 5 de 1917.
Señores Pratt y Cía., agentes de la «Victor Talking Machine Co.»
Estoy muy satisfecho de los nuevos discos «Victor», que he registrado recientemente con mi orquesta.
Puedo asegurar que nunca se ha obtenido tan buen resultado. La pureza, fuerza y claridad del sonido son perfectos, gracias a la excelente calidad del disco «Victor», siendo sorprendente su resultado.
Con mis felicitaciones por el éxito alcanzado, saludo a ustedes muy atentamente,
S. S. S.
E. Arolas
Eduardo Arolas
Véase en la página siguiente la primera lista de estos espléndidos discos.
PIDAN CATALOGOS ILUSTRADOS, GRATIS

Another double page advertisement (28 September 1918) showed Berto, Maglio, Loduca-Canaro, Arolas and the orquestas típicas of Alonso-Minotto and José Arturo Severino, plus 6 non-tango artists.

Nasca and ERA

ERA was a trademark, one of many, used by the Germany-based conglomerate of recording companies, Lindström AG. The financiers in Buenos Aires were the Jacuboff brothers and their front-man entrepreneur was Carlos Nasca who was responsible for selecting local artists, recording and promoting them. Nasca had created for himself a particular persona. He was Italian-born but had completely adopted the cultural heritage of Argentina to such an excessive extent that although living and working in the city he dressed himself as a country gaucho and travelled on horseback, calling himself the 'Gaucho Relampago' (the Lightening Gaucho). He lived alongside his beloved horses all of his life which was suddenly ended aged 63 when one of them delivered to him a fatal kick. Returning to 1911 he formed the Rondalla del Gaucho Relampago and recorded many tangos that we still know today through the recordings of later orchestras, for example *Argañaraz*, *El caburé*, *Una noche de garufa*, *El irresistible*, and the vals *Pabellón de las Rosas*. He also recorded the orquestas típicas of Genaro Espósito and Domingo Biggeri (being quartets of bandoneón, guitar, violin, and flute). Nasca made the recordings at his premises

"ERA"   "ERA"   "ERA"

Nadie se atreverá a negar que los discos de esta marca son los mejores

La rondalla del "Gaucho Relámpago" está siempre por encima de toda competencia.

En venta en las mejores casas de las Repúblicas del Plata.

UNICOS CONCESIONARIOS:

THE INVENTIONS Co.

821, Avenida de Mayo, 823 - Buenos Aires

Importadores de gramófonos, discos y accesorios. - CATALOGOS GRATIS

on the corner of the Avenida Garay and Pirincha and sent the masters to Germany where the discs were manufactured in bulk. A plethora of different labels were applied according to the Buenos Aires customers' wishes. Often the same original recordings appeared under more than one label, including ERA, Phono D'Art, Homokord, Artigas, Chantecler, Beka, and Favorite.

The main retailer of ERA records, The Inventions Company, tried to keep going despite the World War's disruption of trade across the Atlantic. On 9 November 1914 its advertisement added the

38

stoic words that they would continue to trade 'despite the great dangers that the war presents to shipping' but there would be a slight increase in the cost of records. Predictably it could not be sustained and so they looked to the record manufacturers in Brazil and in particular to Saverio Leonetti in Porto Alegre.

The ERA label continued during the war years but who owned it and who was controlling it is opaque, seemingly deliberately so. Recordings emerged bearing the ERA label marked 'manufactured for export by Saverio Leonetti, Porto Alegre'. Tango recordings by the orquestas típicas of Juan Maglio and Felix Camarano also appeared on other labels (Odeon, Phoenix) marked 'recorded by/manufactured for Casa Edison Figner Sao Paolo'. The name of Carlos Nasca is nowhere to be seen and the whole process appears to have been loose, to say the least, and probably involved unauthorised production and copying along the way. Interestingly Leonetti in Porto Alegre produced the record label Gaucho, that was extremely similar in design to ERA's gaucho figure, and Leonetti's tango artists were anonymously named only as 'Orquesta Típica'. Whether the artists benefitted from any of the sales is unknown.

World War I and Brazil

The World War (1914 to 1918) disrupted the European recording industry in general and in particular shipping across the Atlantic. The official statistics[22] for the number of imported discs and cylinders in 1913 was 2,691,000 falling to a mere 276,000 in

---

[22] Dirreción General de Estadísticas de la Nación

1917[23]. However the demand did not diminish. In 1918 the USA trade magazine *Talking Machine World* reported that the demand for talking machines in Argentina and Brazil exceeded supply capacity (due primarily to a post-war shortage of ships) and as a result prices were increasing by 40% as goods were transported on longer rail journeys

The Buenos Aires entrepreneurs who were particularly reliant on German recording engineers and manufacturing plants saw their business models collapse. Alfredo Améndola, Max Glücksmann, and Carlos Nasca found the temporary solution in Brazil.

Fred (Friedrich) Figner was many years ahead of his aspiring Argentinian counterparts. Born in 1866 a hundred kilometres south of Prague he migrated to the USA where he witnessed the wonders of the Edison cylinder phonograph and the moving image camera. He bought models of both and migrated to Brazil in 1892[24] where he began to exhibit them as the new wonders of the modern world. In 1896 he travelled to Buenos Aires to do the same and whilst there created his short films of the Plaza and Avenida de Mayo and scenes from the Palermo gardens. In 1900 he established the Casa Edison in Rio de Janeiro where he not only sold imported Edison products but also made cylinder recordings of local artists. In 1902 Figner negotiated with Zonophone in Germany to host a visiting engineer, Henry Hagen, to record discs[25]. On 15 April 1906 the trade magazine *Talking Machine World* reported that whilst

---

[23] after the war the number of imports never resumed to earlier levels, peaking at less than 500,000, due to the opening of record factories in Buenos Aires (Odeon and Victor)

[24] all references about Figner say 1891 but the passenger list of the ship on which he arrived is dated 1892.

[25] details of the 1902 Zonophone recordings in Buenos Aires are in *Get To Know the Tango Pioneers, Origins to 1909*

Fred Figner used the reputable name of Thomas Edison (his business was Casa Edison) as a marketing tool he mainly dealt with German International Talking Machine and their Odeon discs. By 1911 Figner had the means and the reputation to convince the International Talking Machine company to build a record manufacturing plant under his control in Rio de Janeiro using the name of Odeon. It would soon have the capacity to manufacture 1.5 million discs a year and fortuitously for the South American record industry it was completed in 1913, a year ahead of the start of the World War. It was to Figner and Río de Janeiro that Max Glücksmann turned in 1914. During the war years the volume of records produced for Glucksmann safeguarded the viability of the Rio de Janeiro factory and led to the construction of the manufacturing plant in Buenos Aires (completed in 1920).

In 1908 another immigrant began to make a small mark in the Brazilian music industry. Saverio Leonetti, born 1875 in Italy, set up a store in Porto Alegre selling goods imported from North America and Europe, specialising in electric lamps but also included gramophones and records. Leonetti had his eye on the success of Fred Figner and started re-selling Figner products. On 2 July 1913 he registered the trade mark of his own record label Disco Gaúcho with a detailed description of the label being a colour drawing of a gaucho on horseback (not dissimilar to that of the ERA label). He set up his own basic recording facility and initially sent the masters to Figner in Rio de Janeiro for pressing in to discs until somehow he managed to establish his own disc manufacturing plant. The timing was perfect for both Alfredo Améndola (Atlanta) and Carlos Nasca (ERA) in Buenos Aires who had lost access to their record manufacturers in Germany. Améndola travelled to Porto Alegre with Francisco Canaro, Pedro Polito, and Leopoldo Thompson to record tangos, including

Canaro's latest composition *El chamuyo*. The photograph below was taken in Porto Alegre and shows Leopoldo Thompson standing right, with guitar, next to Francisco Canaro, with violin. Seated are Pedro Polito far left, with his bandoneon, 'Francisco' Schultz (the German recording engineer working for Leonetti), Alfredo Améndola, and to the far right Saverio Leonetti. The names of the flautist and the violinist to the left remain unconfirmed.

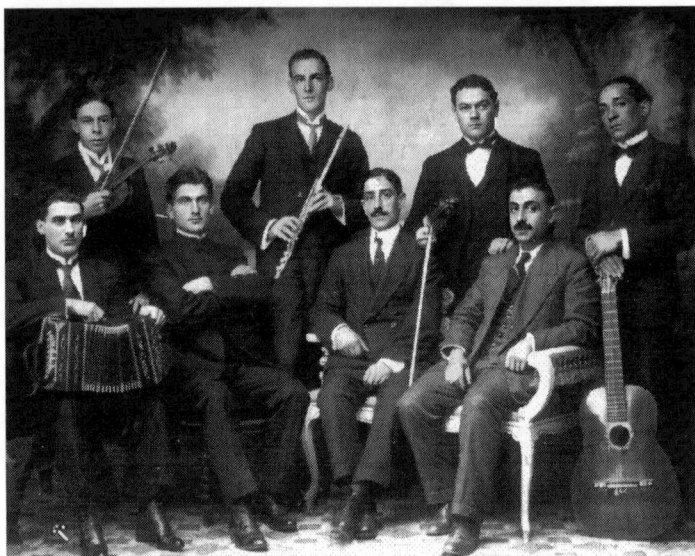

Leonetti also manufactured records by Roberto Firpo, Juan Maglio, Genaro Espósito, and the trio of Juan Carlos Cobían, Osvaldo Fresedo, and Tito Roccatagliata.

2.   Music Sheets

In September 1910 Argentina introduced a law with the intention of protecting the ownership rights of creative works (principally by authors, composers, and inventors) and 12 months later added further protection in the form of criminal sanctions. An examination of the register might suggest that there was a massive creative storm in 1911 but the deluge of entries simply reflects a rush by composers to register and protect their existing back catalogue. Casa Tagini (the Buenos Aires retailer, music publisher, and exclusive agent for Columbia) bombarded the copyright register with its entire catalogue from Columbia. The first tango on the register (on 3 January 1911) was *La rubia* by Ramón Coll but it was not newly composed and had been performed as far back as 1904.

Despite the criminal sanctions, the problem of copyright breaches did not diminish and the financial losses were particularly felt amongst the increasingly prolific tango composers. On 15 October 1918 Francisco Canaro, Francisco Lomuto, Osvaldo Fresedo, Vicente Greco, Augusto Berto, Agustín Bardi, Samuel Castriota, Juan Carlos Bazán, Luis Teisseire, Juan de Dios Filberto, and the publishing company Breyer Brothers formed the Sociedad Nacional de Autores, Compositores y Editores de Música. The Society preceded the 1930 Circle of Authors and Composers of Music that then became, on 9 June 1936 until the present day, the Argentine Association of Authors and Composers of Music (known as SADAIC[26]), initially chaired by Francisco Canaro.

---

[26] Sociedad Argentina de Autores y Compositores de Música

In 1910 Osman Perez Freire (musician, composer, and the grandson of the former Chilean President) produced his monthly *Álbum Musical Centenario* in which he included the musical scores of tangos composed by Rosendo Mendizábal, Alfredo Bevilacqua and others. Whilst promoting those tangos amongst his peers he noticed that although they played the piano well the flow was 'sanitised' in that it had neither the power nor the edge that tango ought to have had. He therefore designed and published his own form of notation in order to help the player correctly interpret the emphasis and rhythm of the city's tango. He was not alone in his discomfort with the mediocre renditions of tango sheet music. On 12 November 1914 the pianist Alfredo Bevilacqua registered the rights to his manual entitled *Escuela del Tango* (Tango School) comprising several piano exercises to help with 22 danceable tangos with particular instruction about getting the correct tango rhythm. Although he dedicated his book to the upper-class Jockey Club (presumably for sponsorship purposes) it was intended to be used by the many middle-class families that had pianos in their homes and who, in his view, were entirely missing the true sense of tango.

In 1913 a Buenos Aires music store published the sheet music for Graciano De Leone's tango *El Rey de la Serpentina* (King of the Parade), a reference to the annual carnival. The elements of bandoneonist Graciano De Leone, a tango, and a carnival all suggest that this was lively music for the ordinary people of Buenos Aires but the drawing on the original sheet music is incongruous: an upper-class drawing room with a lady playing the piano with what may be family members looking on and a young man in waistcoat and bow tie dancing in a side-by-side embrace with his partner. It is evidence that piano sheet music played its role in broadcasting tango to those in the middle and upper-classes, and indicative that the latter tended to play tango demurely to say the least. It is easy to imagine that had he been in the same room Osman Pérez Freire may have become more than a little frustrated with the pace and style of playing.

In a 1915 interview with the magazine *Fray Mocho* the bandoneonist Vicente Greco said that the sheet music sales of his tango composition *El morochito* had reached 22,000 with an unknown additional quantity of pirated copies; his recent *Rodríguez Peña* 12,000; and his latest composition *El Flete* sold 6,000 copies in the first three months of being in the shops. Similarly in a separate interview that year, again in *Fray Mocho,* the bandoneonist Juan Maglio said that the sheet music sales of his first tango composition *El Zurdo* sold 2,000 copies, his second composition *El copetín* about 6,000 and similar amounts for *Armenonville, Casi nada, Adelita,* and *Chile*.

It was clear to all of the tango composers that they were losing substantial revenues of royalty payments due to the widespread sale of illegally copied sheet music. One particular incident illustrates the efforts of the artists themselves to protect their work and the scale of involvement of organised crime in the tango sheet music business. The Sociedad Nacional de Autores, Compositores y Editores de Música laid an information before the magistrate for the Devoto area of Buenos Aires alleging that Miguel Peyret known as 'El Barbún' (due to his trademark long and dishevelled beard) had premises from where he was distributing wholesale consignments to retail outlets. The magistrate authorised a search for suspected counterfeit sheet music and assigned a police officer to accompany the search party that consisted entirely of: the violinist Francisco Canaro, clarinetist Juan Carlos Bazán, flautist Luis Teisseire, and pianists Samuel Castriota, Juan de Dios

Filiberto, and Emilio Iribarne. This group of musicians may not have struck fear in to the hearts of hardened criminals but they certainly had the benefit of motivation. Juan de Dios Filiberto was particularly energised and when frustrated at not finding anything he pushed over what he believed to be barrels of wine in the basement. The barrel lids broke away and the contents were revealed. From all of the barrels they recovered and seized counterfeit music sheets: 250,000 of them.

3.   Pianolas

If you lived in Buenos Aires or Montevideo in 1910, had always wanted to play the piano but had not bothered to learn, had a

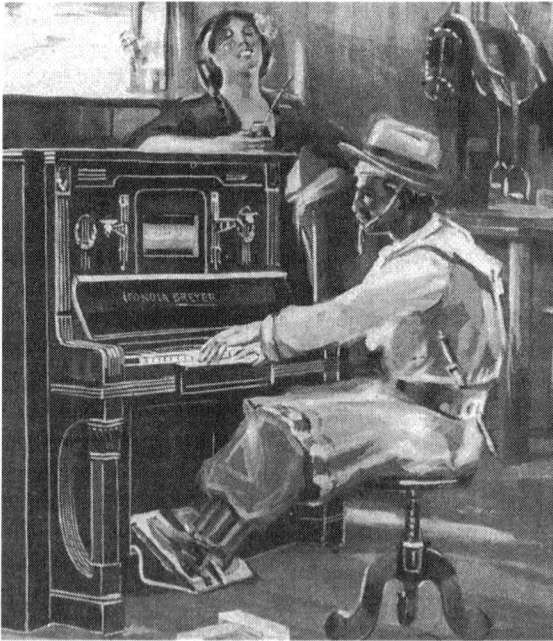

convenient piano-sized space in your parlour and money to spare, then the advertisement in the magazine *La Semana Revista* may have caught your eye: 'pianolas for the modern home that enable everybody to play their favourite pieces without any previous training'. The accompanying pianola rolls included the latest hit tangos.

Developed in the 1890s and first demonstrated in September 1904 in Buenos Aires   (before an audience of 600), these new instruments were modified full-size pianos that could read and play paper rolls punctured with holes that automatically triggered the depression of the keys. It was not entirely automated as the operator needed to ensure the roll turned at a constant speed by using foot pedals (or a wheel) and by making other adjustments by the use of levers.

In June 1910 Max Glücksmann's Casa Lepage advertised the automated Rex piano declaring it to be ideal for owners of bars, confiterias, cinemas, and hotels. The illustration (above), from an advertisement on 1 March 1913, shows a Breyer pianola being played by a country gaucho. The wording says 'without knowing music any person whatsoever can play the piano'.

In 1913 Julio Goossens established a factory manufacturing pianola rolls of Argentinian music, predominantly tango. In order to clearly demonstrate his commitment to national music he branded his rolls as *Pampa*, an acronym for Perforacion Argentina Musical Para Autopianos. After 1913 the manual production of pianola rolls developed in to a system of automation enabling the roll to be mechanically punctured whilst the 'recording' pianist played a piece. Due to the mechanical feed of the roll the finished result was highly unlikely to have captured and reproduced the precise timing played by the recording pianist. Technical staff would therefore amend the roll by adding or removing holes in order to create a regular beat[27]. Although we cannot be sure of the identity of the individual pianist or technician for any particular roll we can be confident that the pianola tango reproductions were as they were played, more or less, by the tango pioneer pianists. Fortunately some were marked as having been recorded directly by a specific pianist, for example a roll for the tango *Chique* is marked as being recorded by the tango pianist and composer Agustín Bardi and bears his signature. Another tango pianist and composer Francisco Lomuto is also known to have produced Pampa rolls. At the piano of Pampa's competitor, Rolla Artis, was Roberto Firpo[28].

Further advances (if technology that replaces a musician can be described as an advance) enabled the production of rolls solely by technicians puncturing all of the holes using a mathematically calculated template on a large piece of graph paper. Most tango pianola rolls that exist today were made between 1913 and 1928.

If you want to recreate the feeling of being at a café-bar in Buenos Aires in the presence of pianists Rosendo Mendizábal, Alfredo Bevilacqua, Manuel Campoamor, Enrique Saborido, Roberto Firpo, Agustín Bardi, or Francisco Lomuto then I highly recommend that you listen to the YouTube Channel videos by my friend Horacio Asborno (pianola collector, restorer and operator) from Viedma, Patagonia.

---

[27] making changes to original recordings (in order to ease the listener's experience) is still a standard practice in today's recording studios

[28] this practice was not limited to tango as famous pianists in the USA to record pianola rolls included George Gershwin and Scott Joplin

4.   Street Organs

Meanwhile the street organs, that were the primary broadcasters of popular tunes prior to 1910, continued to be present and influential in the spread of tangos. In March 1915 a fictional story in *Caras y Caretas* entitled 'El Arrabal' painted the scene of compadritos using the pavement as a dance floor and providing their own music by whistling tangos. It said that whenever there was an

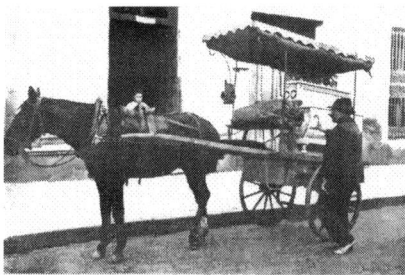

organito[29] present then the whole street came out and got involved in the tango. In 1918 the city authorities banished the wandering organito from (at least) the barrios of El Once, Constitution, and Palermo and on 2 November 1918 *Caras y Caretas* published a sentimental eulogy on the much-loved organito and lamented its ban: 'Wandering the streets the sound captures a sentimental essence, stopping work from all around. In the montonous life of the barrio this heavenly kiss filters through. The organito has passed by but in the souls of the poor the sound of its horns and cylinders remains embalmed'.

The organito in all of its forms from hand-held to horse-drawn was credited with popularising tango across the city. Despite the 1918 ban organitos would continue to be heard on the streets of Buenos Aires for at least a couple of decades more.

---

[29] affectionate name (small organ) for the street organ

5.   Films

The short films of this period (1910 to 1919) began to mirror the themes of the earlier circus and theatre plays celebrating national (creole) culture, for example the 1913 films *Juan Moreira, Tierra Baja,* and *Muerte Civil.* The pioneers of the creole theatre such as Pablo Podestá, Enrique García Velloso, Elías Alippi and José González Castillo were also heavily involved in the new film industry and occasionally used both media at the same time with the overall story being told by actors on the stage together with projected moving images in the background. Those innovations of course drew more people in and made the telling of the creole themes more powerful.

In 1913 Henri 'Enrique' Lepage retired back to his native Belgium and handed over his photography, cinematography, and fonography business to his faithful assistant Max Glücksmann who had joined the Casa Lepage in 1891 aged 16. Almost immediately, on 3 January 1914, Glücksmann secured a three-page article in *Caras y Caretas* focused on his new film empire. That article included photographs of the founder Enrique Lepage, his successor Max, Max's senior managers (his brothers Enrique and Jacobo), and lots of photographs of the outside and inside of their shops, theatres, and

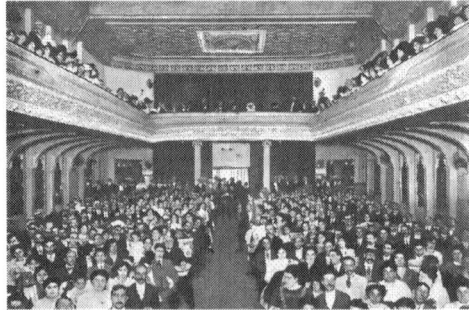

cinemas including the Palace Theatre, El Petit Palace, the Electric Palace, and the Cine Opera. The article was a glowing report on the near monopoly of the Glücksmann film industry. In August of the same year a similar article included a photograph of Glücksmann's luxurious Splendid Teatro with every seat taken for the inauguration of its latest cinema. It was not yet realised but this was the start of the next great broadcasting medium for the promotion of tango.

José Agustín Ferreyra became a prolific maker of Argentinian silent films with a creole theme. Born in Buenos Aires in 1889 and known as El Negro, due to his black Argentinian mother, his speciality was to portray the life of the common people. His film *Nobleza Gaucha*, co-written by José González Castillo, was first shown on 11 August 1915 and opened with a guitar-playing gaucho on horseback. The storyline was the same as the successful themes of the creole circus and theatre, namely a gaucho rescuing a country girl subject to the dishonourable intentions of a wealthy ranch owner at his Buenos Aires property. The film was re-made in 1937 and featured the tango singer Agustín Irusta[30], the musical director was the tango composer and creator of the 1932 milonga rhythm Sebastián Piana, and the script writer was the tango poet Homero Manzi.

In 1916 Ferreyra produced the film *Una Noche de Garufa* and in 1917 *El Tango de la Muerte* with a storyline that has been copied many times in depictions of tango life - the rough working class bar, the seductress, and the tough guy. Another film released in 1916 was *Resaca* (written by José González Castillo based on the play by Alberto Weisbach) set in the tango slums environment in which

---

[30] who recorded with Francisco Canaro from 1927 and 1932

several couples danced tango including the dancer El Cachafez[31] frequently labelled as the best of all tango dancers. In 1917 came the film *La Reina del Tango* about a dissolute woman from the slums who found fame as a tango singer; *Flor de Durazno* in which Carlos Gardel made his, non-singing, film debut; and *Buenos Aires Tenbroso* in which the later tango singer and actress Tita Morello also made her film debut.

Ferreyra, together with pianist Roberto Firpo, had tried valiantly but unsuccessfully to bring synchronised sound (and specifically tango music) to the world of silent films. Films were to stay silent until the start of the 1930s and so prior to that the opening of more and more cinemas meant a demand for musicians to provide the stimulation of sound. Over the coming decade or two those providing the music for silent films included these adolescents:

- pianists Ángel D'Agostino, Rodolfo Biagi, Lucio Demare, and Carlos Di Sarli;
- violinist Juan D'Arienzo; and
- bandoneonists Miguel Caló and Aníbal Troilo

all of whom became leaders of successful tango dance orchestras from the 1930s to the 1950s. Their recordings are heard in every milonga around the world today.

---

[31] Ovidio José Bianquet, born 1885, had a dance school in Buenos Aires in 1913, danced in the USA and Paris and appeared in the 1933 film *Tango*

PART THREE

The Dance

Foreign Tango Mania

On 10 January 1911, the French newspaper *Le Figaro* had correctly foreseen that the most fashionable dance craze of the coming months would be the tango from Argentina. There are a couple of points to draw from this observation:

- it was clear that tango was already established in Argentina and was not in need of a boost from Europe;
- the subsequent European tango mania was for the dance (not the music[32]).

Over the following years newspapers and magazines across Europe regularly reported on the tango dance craze. In February 1913 the Spanish illustrated magazine *Las Ocurrencias* published an article entitled 'The dances that are fashionable in Paris' and showed photographs of couples in the dance holds of the Brazilian Maxixe, the Danza Cubana, the Boston, and the Tango Argentino. Although the photographs all looked similar, the text singled out the tango as the one that was creating a 'real furor in the French high society'. The maxixe dance was also referred to as the Brazilian tango and the Brazilian journalist, former dentist, and self-styled aristocrat 'Monsieur El Duque'[33] claimed in newspapers

---

[32] the interest in tango music was limited to its necessity to support the dance
[33] Antonio Lopes Amorim Diniz

that he had introduced tango to Paris in 1909. To the North Americans and Europeans the maxixe and the tango were similarly exotic from the 'hot Americas' and so the two were often confused, although the simpler word 'tango' was preferable to 'maxixe' and so benefited from more print space. Despite the confusion by commentators the differences between the two were clear. In 1914 Maurice Mouvet (a famed dancer of the French apache, maxixe, and an adapted form of tango) wrote that maxixe could be danced to any 2-step music whilst tango could only be danced to tango music. He added that maxixe was full of 'snap and life' whereas tango was 'slow and languorous'.

<u>Dance Manuals</u>
From 1911 to 1915, before such frivolity petered out during the 1914-1918 World War, dozens of instruction books were published explaining the new tango dance.

In 1911 there were some signs that Parisian tango would follow the Argentine style. Monsieur Robert, the director of the Academy of World Dance in the Rue Pigalle, published *Théorie du Vrai Tango Argentin* (Theory of the True Argentine Tango) in which he recommended that students should only listen and dance to tangos by Argentinian composers (specifically *El choclo* and *El esquinazo* by Villoldo, *Joaquina* by Bergamino, and *Venus* by Bevilacqua) and that they should be danced in a 'very slow rhythm like the habanera'. His reference to the 'true tango' suggests that he already knew that the dance form was being adapted beyond recognition. Most instruction manuals were written by European and North American dance teachers, most of whom are not known to have ever witnessed the social dance in Buenos Aires. Instead they based their instructions and accompanying music on styles that were already familiar to them. The author of *Modern Dancing* (USA 1914) did acknowledge that 'the only drawback in America is that nearly all teachers teach it differently' and he suspected that there was something deeper, a cultural background, to the dance that should not be over-looked: 'it is not only a dance …one must master its style, absorb its atmosphere'.

The manuals were in their own way both authoritative and well-intentioned. Today they help us to understand how the tango dance became so varied to the point of confusion.

Some authors outlined its unsophisticated origins and praised the finesse of the Parisian version:

- *Modern Dancing Simplified* (USA 1914): 'it is danced by the gauchos or cowboys with native women, with bare feet on mother earth. The music is from instruments consisting of a shell containing dried beans, an ordinary piece of wood upon which the drummer taps with a wooden stick….in its original form it could not be possibly danced in a ballroom. But Paris, seeing the possibilities of this beautiful dance, modified it greatly so that we now have the Tango in a very beautiful form';
- *The Secrets of Tango* (England 1914): tango originated 'in the wilds' danced by 'spurred men in heavy boots and the rough maidens of the Argentine country…Parisians advanced the Argentine dance, and handed it back in the shape of a work of art, seductive, charming, and intensely *chic*';
- *Modern Dancing* (USA 1914) admitted that its described tango was a 'sublimated' version, defined as meaning 'modified into a culturally higher, or socially more acceptable, way'.

Others explained that the Argentine tango was far too complex (rather than too unsophisticated) for the non-Argentine dancer:

- *How To Dance The New Dances* (USA 1914): 'The tango as danced in New York is a variation of Argentine Tango. The latter is too complicated for popular usage. The One-Step and the Tango known to the general public are practically twins';

- the *King's Booklet on Dancing* (USA 1914): 'Tango is a name most commonly applied to modern dances but the real tango is seldom danced in the United States. It is a South American folk dance, slow and stately, with many figures of great difficulty. What is called the 'Tango' in this country is really the One Step';

- *How To Dance the Modern Dances* (USA 1914) observed that 'Many descriptions of the Tango have been written, most writers doing little more than illustrating the general confusion and lack of fundamental knowledge regarding the subject. So-called teachers have created steps out of their imagination and called it the Tango. ...The true Argentine Tango is danced by very few people. The Tango is beyond the power of intelligent written description....it demands concentration, intense application and much perseverance'.

Yet even the modified simpler tango carried some warnings of complexity:

- *Modern Dances Tango and Maxixe* (USA 1914) warned that 'it is almost impossible for a gentleman to dance the tango with a lady with whom he has never rehearsed unless both are familiar with the names of the various figures and the gentleman announces in due time to his partner which figures he intends to execute'[34]. Having said that, the author did recognise the value of improvisation: 'if the tango is ever standardised, which I hope it won't be, that would deprive it of much of its beauty and possibilities'.

A few authors seemed disinterested in the Argentine cultural origins and promoted tango simply as light entertainment:

- *The Tango and Turkey Trot* (USA 1913) explained tango in terms of a fitness regime 'above all the Tango is just another name for a beauty exercise' that reduces hips and removes double chins. The author's recommended music was 'the famous tango *Brazilian Dreams'* composed by Will Dixon and the dance steps included 'a kicking step' and on the fourth count 'the couple make a pretty curtsey'. Today's tango dancers will know that none of that makes any sense;

- *How to Dance Tango* (England 1913) said that many dancers had created their own whimsical movements, such as 'the Hen' that involved the foot 'scratching at the floor', the 'Sea Bathing Figure' that involved a dipping movement as if hit by a sudden wave, and 'Sheaves' when travelling rapidly backwards suggesting a long line of wheat sheaves. It appears that the dancers were simply having fun but an Argentinian observer may have thought that they were making fun of their cultural heritage;

- *Practical Guide to Tango and Modern Dances* (USA 1914) detailed several variations under the names of the Maurice Tango, the Joseph Santley Tango, and the Innovation Tango from New York that involved no

---

[34] In contrast today's social dancers are attracted to tango because one can dance with others for the first time and enjoy the improvisation and creativity

contact with the partner and both hands on one's own hips.

From the Argentinian perspective there appeared little enthusiasm for the foreign interpretations:

- in August 1913 the Paris-based Argentinian brothers Alfredo and Armando Guido published their magazine *Mundial* in which they included two drawings showing the difference in dance styles between 'orillero Argentino[35]' and 'aristocratico tango'. They made no specific comment about the differences but I detected in their tone a nostalgia for the 'true' tango from home. The following month the Guido brothers included in their magazine the sheet music of Ángel Villoldo's tango *Elegancia*. The advertisement was headed 'The Tango triumphs everywhere! The celebrated Argentinian composer, the Maestro Villoldo, has just composed his new Tango dedicated to all of the readers of our magazine, *Elegancia* is already creating a storm in all of the Parisian dance schools.' The drawing then showed two ladies dancing together in an embrace with no man in sight. Such images, although not unique to Paris, did come to evoke Parisian tango. In 1913 in Buenos Aires the play *El Tango en París* included a scene of two women dancing tango in a close

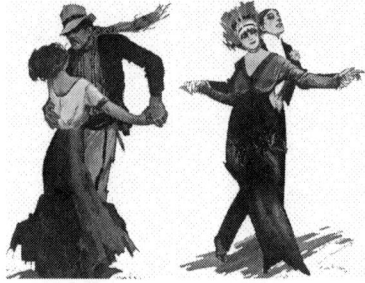

---

[35] meaning from the poorer areas of Buenos Aires

embrace that immediately identified the setting to the audience as Paris.

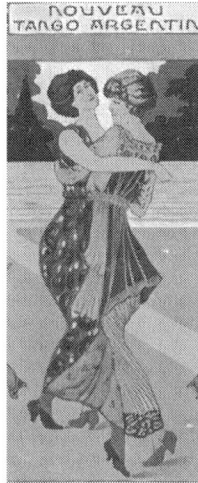

- in December 1913, whilst in Paris, the visiting Argentinian José Salaverría wrote a long article on the dance of tango. He reported that the tango craze was spread across Europe (London, Berlin, Milan, Madrid) and beyond (from New York to St Petersburg). Salaverría marvelled at the power of fashionable trends to dictate the replicated behaviour of men and women across the world, like some form of pandemic. He had seen references to tango in newspapers, in the theatre, on posters and on postcards. It was for that reason that he entered with great expectation in to the salon Olympia to see a tango tea dance in full flow. The room was arranged as he expected: the tables (adorned with tea and cakes) surrounded the central dance floor. Interestingly there were two orchestras that played successively to ensure continuous music that included every conceivable mix of popular genres. But then Salaverría watched with horror as the dancers adopted an exaggerated and graceless style, adding a sense of so-called exoticism to everything they did: the British waltz, the North American Turkey Trot, Grizzly Bear, and Double Boston. Then to his delight the orchestra played tango music but his relief was short lived. The dancers were the same people of course and they threw every effort in to as many rapid contortions as they could muster. He wrote that two women were dancing together who, as they had no idea how to dance, just simply invented random movements. Salaverría was left completely confused how this tango, that was definitely not the tango that he knew from Buenos Aires, could have become so fervently popular. He described his indignation at the scene 'oh poor tango how they have removed all your passion and elegance of the common people'. He did accept that he may have just been unlucky in his choice of venue – today's reader who is a well-travelled tango dancer may recognise that experience;

- in 1914 the Argentinian tango dancer Juan Barrasa[36], based in London, said that real tango is infinitely better adapted to the ballroom than the spurious inventions of London and Paris. It seems that he had endured similar experiences to those of his countryman Salaverría.

---

[36] a wealthy son of a landowner in the provinces of Argentina

Meanwhile in Buenos Aires the press had been reporting on what was happening to their national culture:

- in 1912 the newspaper *El Diario* stated "...the tango that is danced in Paris isn't ours more than the name and the music...it isn't more than a rough imitation of 'our' tango";

- on 3 May 1912 the magazine *Fray Mocho* reproduced an article from the British magazine, *The Sketch*, that had celebrated the successful production of 'tango argentino' at the London Gaeity theatre. *Fray Mocho* mockingly entitled it 'Overseas Fantasy' (below);

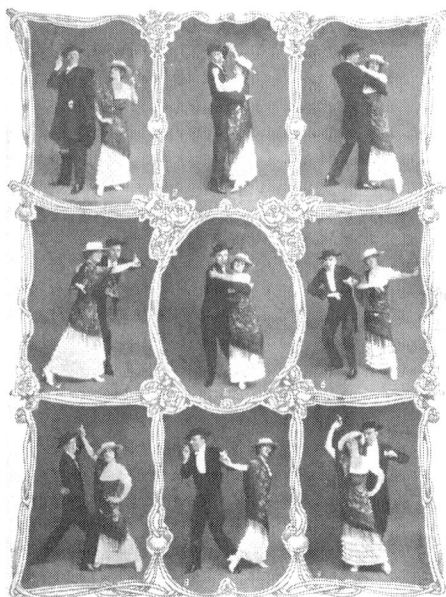

El tango argentino en el Gaety de Londres

1. El comienzo, 2. empieza el baile, 3. la primera vuelta, 4. el tercer movimiento, 5. la cuarta, 6. una variación de la corrida, 7. al sexto movimiento, 8. el séptimo movimiento, el "gaucho de los pies", 9. Figura final

- On 20 August 1912, the Buenos Aires magazine *Sherlock Holmes* published an article entitled 'La muerte del Tango' (the death of tango). It blamed Paris for killing tango, describing (in far too many similar analogies) how tango, the poor overseas adventurer, ended up asphyxiated by the boudoir perfumes of France;

- On 3 January 1914 *Caras y Caretas* published a page entitled 'Tangomania in Europe' (below).

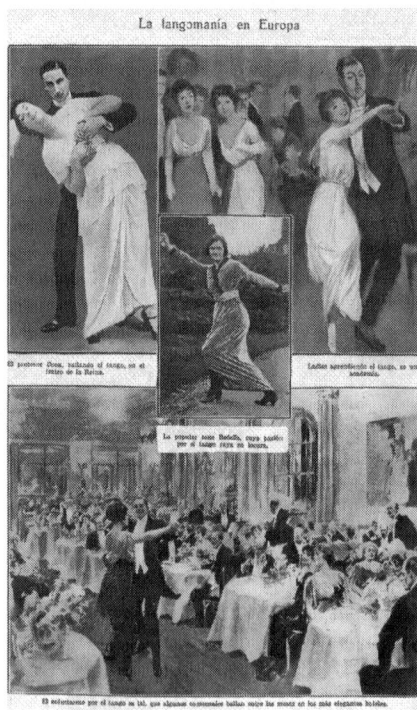

La tangomanía en Europa

If you want to study the detailed step by step instructions for tango in Europe and the USA between 1911 and 1915 then I refer you to the Library of Dance website[37] where you can find many of the manuals including diagrams and photographs. If you prefer light entertainment I can recommend a short film *Max, Professeur de Tango*[38]. In February 1914 the French comedy actor Max Linder released a film (made two years earlier in Berlin) about a drunken teacher of tango. Max Linder was not a tango dancer nor particularly interested in tango, the film was simply one of hundreds of similar slapstick shorts that by 1914 had elevated him to the position of best-paid film star in the world. The film does however give us a comical insight in to the world of European upper-class tangomania.

The Dance Music
Tango mania was for the dance not the music, but music was necessary. There were Argentinian tango musicians in Europe and the USA but they:

- were too few to influence the national scene;
- adapted their style to suit the national audiences;
- were supplemented by local musicians unfamiliar with Argentine tango;
- were themselves not necessarily representative of the music scene back in Buenos Aires.

---

[37] https://www.libraryofdance.org/dances/early-tango/
[38] available on YouTube

Each country's dance band musicians played in their own familiar style and on familiar instruments. They played the tangos for which they had the sheet music and the vast majority of available sheet music came from European and North American composers. The resulting sound was therefore very different from tango music in Argentina. The most commonly played Argentinian tangos were *El choclo*, *El esquinazo*, *El irresistible*, *Joaquina*, and *Venus* – not because they were judged to have been the best but because they had the most readily available sheet music.

The dance manual *How to Dance Tango* (1913 England) included a chapter dedicated to 'Tango Music'. The author[39] said that composers, printers of sheet music, and 'gramophone-record makers' could not keep up with the demand but were nevertheless earning a fortune. The recommended European and North American composers and their most popular tangos have now faded into obscurity but those from Argentina (Villoldo's *El choclo*, Logatti's *El irresistible*, and Begamino's *Joaquina*) still remain favourites today. Regardless of which tango was played the author stressed that the most important factor was the strong bass 'which presents difficulties to even the really skilled pianist unless a very powerful player'. To that end she recommended her readers to hire a pianola, particularly with the rolls for *El choclo*, *Joaquina*, *Apollo* and *Venus*.

In 1914 the the author of *The Secrets of Tango* interviewed London-based Argentinian tango dancer Juan Barras who recommended the Argentinian tangos *Joaquina*, *El esquinazo*, and *El irresistible.*

---

[39] amongst the long list of male authors and dance instructors was Gladys Beattie Crozier, London. A prolific writer of articles for the *Ladies Review* including in September 1905 *Practical Motoring for Ladies*

In 1914 the Victor Talking Machine company published a couple of free guides entitled *3 Modern Dances*. As well as the detailed descriptions of dance steps the guides recommended records for dancing tango. In one guide none of the recommended tangos were by Argentinian composers and all were recorded by the USA Military Band. The other Victor guide did at least include *Argañarez, Didi* and *El amanecer* (composed by Roberto Firpo) but they were again played by Victor's own North American bands. In contrast, during the same year, the Columbia Graphophone Company produced its own free guide *How to Dance the Modern Dances* and said that 'very little suitable tango music has been written by (North) American composers'. It recommended its tango records by Argentinian composers Villoldo, De Bassi, and Gobbi that had been recorded in Buenos Aires by the city's Municipal Band.

There were dozens of versions of Argentinian tangos recorded across Europe and the USA for the dancer, for example:

- *El choclo* (by Villoldo) in 1912 by a brass band recorded in Vilnius on the Zonophone label and by the Victor Orchestra in New Jersey; in 1913 by the National Promenade Band in New York on the Edison label and by the Orchester des Palais de Danse in Berlin;
- *El irresistible* (by Logatti) in 1913 by the Gramophon Orchestra in Moscow; by Europe's Society Orchestra in New York; and the Orchestre Tzigane in Paris;
- *Joaquina* (by Bergamino) in 1910 by the Victor Orchestra New Jersey; in 1913 by the Hungarian Gypsy String Orchestra in Warsaw; and in 1914 by the Orchestre Tzigane in Paris;
- *El Argentino* and *El esquinazo* (by Villoldo) in 1913 by the Moulin Rouge Orchester in Berlin;

- *Apollo* (by Bevilacqua) in 1913 by the Orchester Pederetti Vom Residenz Café in Berlin;
- *Don Juan* (by Villoldo) in 1913 by the Orchestre Tzigane in Paris; and
- *La catrera* (by De Bassi) also in 1913 Paris by the Orchestre Tzigane.

The War

Tango mania raged from 1911 to 1914 and understandably diminished from 1915 to 1919 due to the social and economic upheaval of the World War. In 1915 a cartoon in a French newspaper captured the sudden change in circumstance and mood. The cartoon consisted of two frames: in the first were tango dancers with the commentary 'a little more than a year ago she danced tango and was incapable of thinking of anything else'; and the second showed a nurse attending a wounded patient 'how she was mistaken! That young girl with such dedication now cares for the injured'. Another in 1917 was dedicated to the young girls of France: 'farewell to tennis, flirting, and the tango teas. Yesterday frivolity, today courage'. And in 1919 an article celebrated 'The youth return to dance'. But it was not as before – the tango was too solemn and the appetite was for joyous music, provided by the North American fox-trot.

A new flurry of dance manuals were published in 1922 in the USA:

- *Dancing Made Easy* provided fulsome explanations of all of the popular dances and, in passing, stated that 'the tango has succumbed to the antidote of dances

> that are more sensible and easily learned. Supreme of these is the Fox Trot'; and

- *The Modern Dances* by the Arthur Murray School of Dancing made no mention of tango at all.

In Europe and North America the dance and music of Argentinian tango was to fall from fashion[40].

In Argentina

The tango dance of the opening decades of the twentieth century is nearly always portrayed in two starkly contrasting ways:

- the coarse movements of the compaditos (the lower classes) that was rejected by decent society; and
- the anodyne style of the aristocracy that was mocked for its faux-Parisian airs.

Those styles of dancing did exist at either end of the social scale but we have been left with little sense of how the majority of the population danced tango because, unlike in Europe and North America, tango did not burst on to the scene in a peak of fashionable frenzy and so did not attract volumes of documentary evidence. I was therefore delighted to unearth several revealing sources.

Dance Manuals

Nicanor M. Lima published in 1914 *El Tango Argentino de Salon, Metodo de Baile, Teorico y Practico* (Argentine Tango for the Dance Floor, Method of Dance, Theory and Practice). This was not commercially motivated to cash in on the latest modern dance

---

[40] See *Get To Know the Tango Pioneers: 1920 to 1935 the Precarious Years*

craze because tango was not new. It is clear to me that Lima had studied the dance over many years and felt the need to re-assert its cultural importance.

> *Tango Argentino is a national dance, it is our very soul…it is an artistic dance that requires of its proponents the maximum grace, elegance, and rhythm. Its music is so sentimental and beautiful that we cannot hear it impassively without becoming part of its symphony, without accompanying it with movement, without fully concentrating on it, and without imagining a dance salon full of couples elegeantly dancing its many beautiful and difficult figures.*

He shows us that tango was not a coarse degenerate sub-culture, nor a passing fashion, and certainly not an adoption of the Parisian tangomania. Argentine tango was a national dance and was in the soul of the people. That means it had been around for a long time and was widely spread. But who were the people in whose soul it lay? The drawings of the dancing couple on the cover and throughout the manual were shown in smart clothing of the middle classes. The man was wearing a sombre jacket and tie (neither an upper-class dinner jacket with bow tie nor the compadrito's hat, scarf and thick-heeled shoes). The lady was in a modest full-length skirt, neither an elegant gown nor a revealing dress.

Dermidio T. Gonzalez, a poet and author of Argentinian history, wrote the prologue to the manual. He too was a promoter of Argentinean tango danced with the 'cuteness, elegance, honesty and simplicity that characterizes our graceful Creoles'. He praised Nicanor Lima's efforts to ensure that 'tango occupies the place it deserves amongst our country's most beautiful traditions'.

In the body of the manual Lima made four overarching points:

- it was all about the embrace: 'there is never a case in which the couple can separate or release each other, dancing alone or solo';
- and the music: 'hence the music will facilitate very much the learning of the dance';
- it was not about the figures: 'It is the case that in the other hemisphere (Europe), and even in our own country, that in our labours to create many diverse steps, many have applied to our beautiful dance whichever capricious little silly thing imaginable, making the posture of the couple, and in the end, the dance itself, ridiculous';
- Argentine tango was the true tango: 'there is no Parisian Tango, and if there were, it would only be a degenerate copy of the Argentine Tango'.

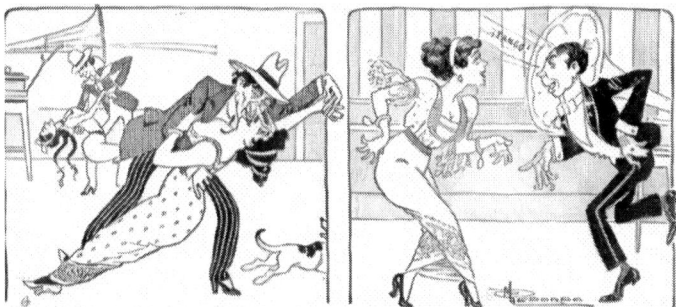

This Buenos Aires cartoon from 1912 showed the sort of dance behaviour that may have inspired Lima to re-set the dial. On the left the music being played from the gramophone is described as a vals but the compadritos are dancing their extreme tango style whilst on the right the upper class couple are dancing the cake-walk to tango music. I make no apology for repeating myself when

I say that tango cannot be defined, nor explained, as it is and has always been so many different things to different people.

A technical note for tango dancers Nicanor Lima's manual provides extensive detail about dance moves, many of which are still familiar to today's dancers. Of particular note is that they are all in the parallel system including the ochos (forward and back). The cross system was not developed until the 1940s[41].

A further insight in to the Argentinian dancing style of tango comes from the Spanish author Enrique Gómez Carillo who spent a month in 1914 in Buenos Aires and kept extensive notes of his experiences in the city. Over the following 5 years he returned several times and extended his journals in to a book that he completed and published in Madrid in 1921. The title was *El Encanto de Buenos Aires* (The Charm of Buenos Aires) and he dedicated one short chapter to tango. With two friends and a local guide he visited a dance hall in the working-class dockside barrio of La Boca. His guide had warned him to expect coarse people, behaviour, and dancing that was a world away from what he may have witnessed in Paris. They entered the large unadorned room, dark with few gaslights where perhaps a hundred locals were chatting, laughing, and drinking. The men, mainly young, were wearing bowler hats and with the demeanour of what he knew to be called 'compadritos'. The women seemed to represent the wider female population from the very young to the old but those that Enrique particularly noticed, and found somewhat unsettling, were those whose eyes fixed on every man that entered the room with a

---

[41] Parallel system: the leader and follower are stepping with legs opposite each other (mirroring each other's steps). Cross system: the leader and follower are using the same foot at each step (their right at the same time or left at the same time).

challenging and provocative smile. In today's tango dance halls this is known as the *mirada* (the look) and precedes the mutually agreed contract to dance. He felt safer just to sit and watch the dancing. The couples passed by, one after the other in a line, with neither rushed nor harsh movements, and taking care of their steps in a lightly-held embrace. Their faces were serene, paradoxically serious and smiling. Despite his surroundings he could see no difference between the tango in La Boca and the tango in the finest tea dances in Paris. He strongly disputed the allegations of the dance's impropriety (made by the Argentina Ambassador to France, Rodriguez Larreta[42]) and wrote: "tango Argentino is a dance that is slow, elegant, distinguished, aristocratic, complicated and chaste....there is not a single movement that the most purest of ladies could not do". Enrique was bemused where this mistaken view had all come from - had the Parisian refinement somehow reached this distant and, quite frankly, miserable joint in La Boca? He knew that the dance had nothing in common with the shocks, shakes, tensions, and pantomine of the tango andaluz[43]. Nor could he believe that the dance he was witnessing came from the ranch workers of the pampa nor from the sailors in brothels - "that is what the people believe because the newspapers say so. But I cannot logically accept it." Today there is widespread confusion about the origins and development of tango but thanks to Enrique Gómez Carillo we now know that our picture is not clear because it had never been clear.

Before we move on, he also told us something of the music that inspired the dancers that night in La Boca. It was a sextet. The violins (powerful, subtle, and languid) delivered the delicious tango

---

[42] 'the tango in Buenos Aires is a dance exclusive to brothels and bars of the worst kind'. See *Get To Know the Tango Pioneers Origins to 1909*
[43] his description not mine

rhythm that was so familiar to him from Paris. He said no more but we can make an assumption: being a sextet at that time in all likelihood it would have consisted of two violins, two bandoneóns, a piano, and a double bass. That was a serious formation pre-1920 and I would not be surprised if the musicians that evening included some of those featured in the Pioneer sections in Part Four below.

Other insights in to Argentinian dance events appeared in newspapers although (being part of everyday social life) they attracted scant attention. One report in April 1912 allows us a peek in to a social club for ordinary folk. Cayetano Ganghi, a key figure in the political party Unión Cívica Radical (UCR)[44], organised a tango dance competition at the Club Carlos Pellegrini in order to rally support for the March 1912 elections. The prizes for the best tango and the best vals were cash prizes for the men and gold bracelets for the women (although the women were massively under-represented in the published photograph.

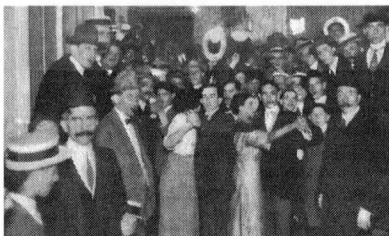

In June and July 1914 the Inventions Company, on the Avenida de Mayo, advertised its collection of ERA records. That was not unusual but on those occasions it used drawn images and descriptions of the tango dance. One headed 'el tango criollo' showed a working-class couple, the woman wearing an apron and a shawl; another showed a middle-class couple, the man wearing a

---

[44] the UCR represented the working-class population and is celebrated by several tangos. Those best-known today include *Unión Cívica* recorded by Juan D'Arienzo and by Rodolfo Biagi (both in 1938)

suit and straw hat with the words 'Vd tanguea?' (do you dance tango?); the third was of an upper-class couple, the man wearing a tail coat and bow tie and the text said 'Without tango, life is not worth the trouble. Dance tango and be happy, especially in these cold days of financial difficulties. If you have a fonograph then follow our advice and dance tango whenever you can'. Their record selection of tango dance tunes was the same for everyone regardless of social classes. The same tango music and dance belonged to everyone, even children.

On 29 September 1917 *Caras y Caretas* published a photograph of a group of school children outdoors, two in a close embrace, and an adult was playing a gramophone record. The photograph was annotated 'during break between lessons dancing tango to the rhythm of the fonograph'. Unfortunately the names of neither the recorded artists nor the tango track were identified.

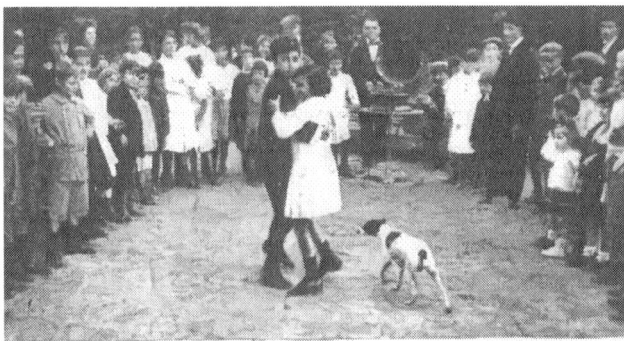

Intermezzo obligado. — Bailando un tango al compás del fonógrafo.

Part Three   Dance

PART FOUR

The Tango Pioneers

*Dancers, singers,
pianists, bandoneonists, violinists,
flautists, guitarists*

1. Dancers

During the decade 1910 to 1919 a few young men from wealthy Argentinian families (who had been involved in the tango scene in Buenos Aires) went to Paris to enjoy the fashionable high life. Whilst there they danced and taught tango.

Ricardo Güiraldes, born in 1888, had travelled between Argentina and Europe as a child with his family and so the idea of going to Paris in 1909, aged 23, was neither an unusual nor particularly adventurous thing for him to do. He easily convinced his friend Daniel Dorna to accompany him. They demonstrated their tango dance to the high society of Paris, each having their own distinctive style. Güiraldes was energetic and liked to demonstrate figures whereas Dorna preferred to glide and to perfect his undecorated walk. Today's tango dancers will recognise these styles at both ends of the tango dance spectrum.

Meanwhile in 1910 back in Buenos Aires the tango teacher Bernabé Simarra (right) was giving lessons to the visiting French actress, Mademoiselle Papillon, who then paid for him to return with her to Paris. Once there, not only did Simarra continue to teach the rich and famous but he also took to the stage and became widely known as 'The King of Tango', ostentatiously dressed in exaggerated gaucho clothes including spurs. It is not surprising that today's images of tango are so diverse and confusing

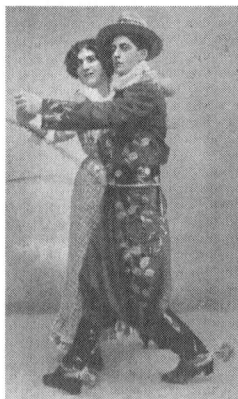

because tango was forever thus - many things to many people. Simarra became a tango dancing celebrity amongst high society in France, Italy, and Spain but his comfortable retirement unravelled dismally during the Spanish Civil War. He was forced to abandon his home and possessions in 1936 and ended his days, unknown and impecunious, in Uruguay.

On 11 July 1911 the Buenos Aires magazine *Sherlock Holmes* reported on the success of the locally born Francisco Ducasse who was 'discovered' at a Parisian café whistling the tango *El Caburé* and dancing alone. He subsequently won first prize in a high society dance competition and was subsequently taken in to the hearts and homes of the rich and famous. Ducasse returned to Buenos Aires and featured in the magazine *Fray Mocho* (13 February 1914) that dedicated two pages to 'How to dance tango in Argentina' including photographs of Ducasse in various dance positions with the actress Blanca Podestá[45], together with feet placement diagrams and explanations. The article added that Ducasse was 'one of our best tango dancers' who deservedly won first prize whilst dancing with Princess Murat in a competition in the Femina theatre, Paris. The journalist may have intentionally undermined that accolade when he described Parisian tango as containing undecipherable postures that make our own (Argentinian) dancers both laugh and protest.

Ovidio José Bianquet, known as El Cachafaz, was born in 1885. He had made a name for himself in the dance halls of Buenos Aires and in 1912 travelled as part of a theatrical troupe to the USA as the partner to a famous tango dancer of the day, Eloisa

---

[45] of the famous circus and theatre family, see *Get To Know the Tango Pioneers Origins to 1909*

Gabbi[46]. He returned in 1913 and opened a tango dance academy, spent a short time in 1919 demonstrating and teaching in Paris, and preserved his place in history by appearing in the films *Resaca (1916)* and particularly in *Tango* (1933) in which he danced to the tango *El Entrerriano*.

In 1912 the aristocratic Antonio María De Marchi organised a tango event at the recently opened Palais de Glace[47] in Buenos Aires. He invited Enrique Saborido (the renowned tango pianist and composer) as the performing dancer who by that time had also established his own dance academy. The event was entirely inspired by the Parisian tango scene and within a few months Saborido travelled to France. Saborido's hosts, and sponsors, were members of the French aristocracy, principally Madame de Reszké and Baron Henri de Rothschild. By the time Saborido arrived the national newspaper *Le Gaulois* was already reporting almost daily on high society tango dance events and competitions, at which were often (different) 'Kings of Tango'. On 9 February 1914 it reported on yet another high society event at which the latest 'King of Tango', Saborido, demonstrated the new dance.

In 1913 the magazine *Sherlock Holmes* published, in two successive weeks, multiple-page articles on the dance academy of Casimiro Ain, that had been trading as 'Cain y Abel' for two years. The first

---

[46] the North American newspapers reported the great dancer Eloisa Gabbi but made only passing mention of 'her assistant' Bianquet.

[47] De Marchi is often named as an influential aristocratic figure in the development of tango in Buenos Aires in 1912/13. There is no primary evidence to support the repeated claim that he promoted orquestas típicas amongst the upper-classes. There is evidence that his tango extravaganza on 22 September 1913 at the Palace Theatre on the Calle Corrientes involved music by the classical cellist Carlos Marchal and the prize for the best tango composition went to a French-born landowner from La Pampa.

article on 22 April included six photographs of the owner Ain and his associate dance instructor Eduardo Reus dancing together. Photographs also showed them both in turn dancing with the academy's female teacher Ema Ramos. The journalist had entered the city centre café where a tango quartet was playing and he descended in to the basement to find that a class was underway. Casimiro Ain told him that he had 70 couples as students and the previous year he had taught 190 men including those from the upper echelons of society. He further revealed that he was imminently going to Paris with the music trio of Vicente Loduca to set up a dance academy. The contract had been arranged by the Argentinian Alberto López Buchardo who had established himself in Paris in 1906 as a tango dancer, teacher, pianist, and composer. And sure enough only two months later, on 26 June 1913, the French newspaper *Le Figaro* reported the appearance at the Moulin Rouge of an Argentine troupe - the 'recently arrived dancers Casimiro Ain and his wife Marta (also known as Martina) and the musicians Loduca, Ferrer, and Monelos'. They shared the stage with the already famous Argentinian dancer Bernabé Simarra and in July they were at the Folies Bergère performing in a show called 'A night in Buenos Aires'. Later that year Casimiro & Marta Ain, Loduca, Ferrer, and Monelos travelled by invitation to New York. In March 1914 the magazine *Fray Mocho* described them as the troupe of Ain-Loduca, placing the name of the dancer first and the bandoneonist second.

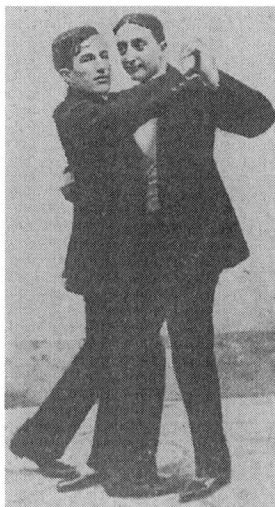

Ain then returned to Paris, with pianist Ferrer, and joined together with recently arrived bandoneonist Güerino Filipotto and violinist José Sentio in July 1914 to perform at the Café Argentina and other Parisian venues. At the same time Germany declared war on France and the First World War began. Ain and his wife soon departed Europe for Argentina and after the war had finished he visited Paris again, in 1920, but by that time he had found a new partner, Edith Peggy.

On 20 July 1912, the magazine *Caras y Caretas* published a three-page article entitled 'The Success of Tango'. The overall purpose of the article was to note how the humble tango from the Buenos Aires slum outskirts[48] had established itself in the best dance salons of fashionable Paris and London. It noted that the appetite of the European upper-classes for Argentinian tango lessons had exceeded the capacity of the relatively few visiting Argentinians to such an extent that even lower-class Argentinians (that the article did not name) had travelled to Paris and transformed themselves in to the darlings of the rich. However, it seems that not all visiting Argentinian dance teachers were automatically successful. On 6 September 1913 the same magazine carried a full-page cartoon entitled 'El professor de tango de Buenos Aires a Paris y vice versa'. It showed the impoverished porteño earning his cheap sea passage to Paris, advertising tango lessons, and then becoming so successful that he invited others over to work for him in order to meet the ever-increasing demand. He discovered that his assistants had set up their own schools, leaving him without any business. He returned penniless to Buenos Aires and was last seen peeling potatoes as an unskilled kitchen worker. Like all good cartoons it

---

[48] this line suggests the origins to have been from the slums but the evidence demonstrates otherwise, see *Get To Know the Tango Pioneers, Origins to 1909*

would have resonated with its readers who must have recognised similar situations. Today it reminds us that there are always many more personal experiences behind the more frequently told successful highlights.

The pressure on visting Argentinans to show their tango skills was not only on the teachers but also on the travelling high society. All of those sailing to Paris whether for pleasure or business, being Argentinian, were expected to dance tango and to dance it well. Thankfully for them Juan Carlos Herrera, who described himself as a 'doctor in tangology', opened a dance academy on the Avenida Bartolomé Mitre (midway between today's Obelisco and the Plaza de Congreso). For those who could not yet dance tango and wanted instant results he promised to teach in only a few lessons a series of eye-catching decorative steps including the adventurous quebrada. On 9 August 1913 *Caras y Caretas* published photographs of Herrera and a class of pre-travel students (below) and the following month he was listed as a notable contestant in a tango dance competition at the Sociedad Sportiva. In 1914 the

refined tango pianist and composer Juan Carlos Cobían abandoned his down-market tango lifestyle in order to be Herrera's dance studio pianist - a

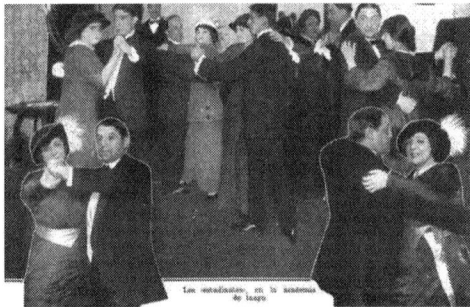

Los estudiantes en la academia de tango

much happier environment for him, playing tango in the company of sophisticated and wealthy clients.

2. The Singers

Bianco, Contursi, Gardel, Mathón,
Membrives

Francisco Bianco

Francisco Bianco was a folk singer, lyricist and composer who crossed paths with the emerging tango stars and introduced his lyrics and voice in to their instrumentals. Unusually for singers at that time his voice did not transform the tango in to a ballad (for sitting and listening) but perfectly kept the dancing rhythm. He was the pioneer of the tango singer for the dance floor.

He was born in 1894 in the city of Rosario, Argentina, but the family moved to Buenos Aires shortly afterwards. His father was the director of a music school, played in an orchestra, and taught Francisco and his older brother Eduardo[49] how to read music and play instruments. In 1902 Francisco's mother rented out a room to the French immigrants Berthe Gardès and her young son Charles. The two boys became friends and both grew up to play guitar and sing national creole songs: Charles Gardès transformed

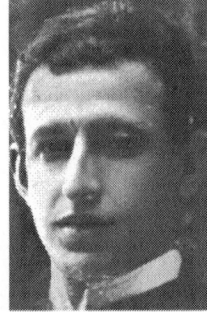

---

[49] Eduardo Bianco, a violinist made his fame as tango composer and orchestra leader in Europe from the 1920s to 1943

in to the world famous Carlos Gardel whilst Francisco's name today is barely known.

Bianco started performing professionally in 1909 and by the age of 19 he had become a prolific and respected lyricist and singer. In 1913 he toured with the most famous payadors including Gabino Ezeiza, Ambrosio Ríos, and José Betinotti and that year made 10 recordings of folk songs on the Columbia label. In 1914 his verses were published in *Songs of the Soul - songs of Francisco Nicolas Bianco* and his subsequent popularity earned him a long-standing recording contract on the ERA label.

In February 1917 in the magazine *Fray Mocho*[50] he lamented that although he still attracted large audiences in the provinces there was a fading interest in his style in Buenos Aires itself. He did not venture a reason for the change in the city's musical preferences but by then he had already started to work together with some of the tango bandoneonists, presumably in acknowledgment of where that new interest lay. On 15 May Francisco Bianco was in the temporary studio set up by the visiting Victor engineers George Cheney and Charles Althouse. He was there to sing lyrics to the tango *La payanca*, accompanied by the popular Eduardo Arolas quintet, but it was not a great day for Bianco. He spoiled his first take of *La payanca* – the engineers noted 'singer choked at beginning of second verse' and he had to re-take it. It is now an excellent and rare example of a danceable, sung tango from the era of acoustic recordings. On the next recording, the vals *El aeroplano*, (also an excellent danceable recording) they noted that there were 'two break-downs on good blanks'. It is not clear whether the

---

[50] the article described him as 'the veteran singer and creole lyricist' even though he had just turned 23.

breakdown was mechanical or human but either way they lamented the waste of blank master discs. After another two recordings (of Arolas instrumentals) Francisco Bianco came back in to the room to record *Dolorido* but during that session the engineers' patience had run out 'Breakdown - came in too early- did same thing in test'. Bianco was not on top form. Cheney and Althouse took great care with the arrangement of the instruments in the room to ensure a balanced sound and all was going well until Bianco moved too close to the recording horn. In the second take Bianco had not made any mistakes and then just before the recording had finished the 'second violinist spoke'[51]. The third take was no better leading to an exasperated entry 'Punishment?' and no further recordings were attempted that day.

Many tango commentators describe the recording as 'Arolas with Francisco Bianco' suggesting that the singer had a secondary role but when it was advertised on 8 December 1917 the disc was promoted with Bianco's photograph rather than that of Arolas. The star attraction was most definitely Francisco Bianco. He then recorded at Nacional Odeon supported by the resident orchestra of pianist Roberto Firpo. Although he had expanded his appeal to the new popular tango dance market his heart and his future remained in the poetry and song of the national creole folk genre, just as it would for Carlos Gardel in the years ahead. Bianco was also affectionately known as Pancho Cuevas.

You can also hear the lyrics of Bianco in the vals *Ausencia* recorded by Carlos Di Sarli (1940) and Francisco Canaro (1949).

---

[51] the violinists were Carlos Lombardo and Rafael Tuegols

Pascual Contursi

Pascual Contursi was a folk singer/guitarist who made his mark in the history of tango as the lyricist of one tango: *Mi noche triste*, declared by many to have been the first *tango canción*[52].

Contursi was born in 1888 and raised in the provinces some 160 kilometres inland from Buenos Aires. Having first moved with his family to Buenos Aires he decided as a young man that he preferred to live in Uruguay. On 22 March 1916 the Montevideo newspaper *El Día* reported that the young creole singer/guitarist Pascual Contursi was performing at the Moulin Rouge cabaret. He sang and played requests from the audience that included the repertoire of the duo Gardel-Razzano[53] together with well-known tunes to which he had added his own lyrics. One of those that was well-received was his sung rendition of the tango *El flete*, composed as an instrumental by bandoneonist Vicente Greco. Contursi also added his own lyrics (and his own titles) to the compositions of Eduardo Arolas (*La guitarrita*), Manuel Aróztegui (*Champagne tango*), and others.

In Buenos Aires in 1916 the pianist Samuel Castriota published the sheet music to his tango composition *Lita*[54]. In his usual manner Pascual Contursi penned words to *Lita* without any reference to, and certainly not approval from, the composer Castriota. Contursi managed to

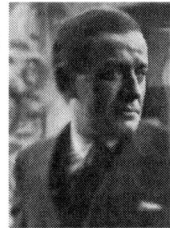

---

[52] A tango that tells a structured story, usually emotional

[53] That did not include tangos at that time

[54] That has subsequently found to have been heavily influenced by an earlier 1914 melody

get his version of the tango to Carlos Gardel who liked it and tested it in front of his friends who also approved. In April 1917, at the premises of Max Glücksmann's Nacional Odeon, the duo Gardel-Razzano recorded it as the re-named *Mi noche triste* (as a B-side to a zamba) and the label credited both Castriota (composer) and Contursi (lyricist). A few days later Glücksmann's other leading artist Roberto Firpo recorded an instrumental version for the dance floor and, being without lyrics, the label only credited Samuel Castriota. Despite being recorded by two of the most successful artists the tango *Mi noche triste* was initially received with little or no acclaim.

In 1918 the production team of the play *Los dientes del perro* was looking for a tango to be played, set in a cabaret. They chose *Mi noche triste* that was performed by the orquesta típica of Roberto Firpo and sung by the actress Manolita Poli (right). The play was a huge success and included *Mi noche triste* for over 400 performances until it was withdrawn due to a dispute following Contursi's demand to be paid 50% of the royalties. It was certainly the lyrics rather than the music that had caused a public stir. On 29 June 1918 the magazine *El Teatro Nacional* published the lyrics in full thereby reaching more than the theatre's audience. However there were several other reasons that contributed to the play's success:

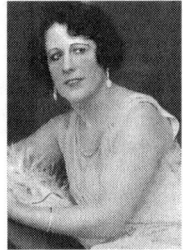

- Manolita Poli's performance (irrespective of the construction or lyrics of the song);
- for the first time an orquesta típica was on stage as part of the storyline in a cabaret (as opposed to being in the orchestra pit); and
- the orchestra was that of the famous Roberto Firpo.

Mi noche triste was subsequently recorded by many artists including: Alberto Gómez (1932), Francisco Canaro with Roberto Maida (1936), Osvaldo Fresedo with Oscar Serpa (1942), and Aníbal Troilo with Edmundo Rivero (1949).

Pascual Contursi achieved limited success thereafter but we shall meet him again briefly in *Get To Know the Tango Pioneers 1920 to 1935* together with his son José Maria Contursi who achieved greater success than his father as a tango lyricist.

Carlos Gardel

On 12 February 1893 at the dockside of Bordeaux, France the unmarried mother Marie Berthe Gardès Camarès boarded the ship *Don Pedro* for a journey across the Atlantic to South America. In her arms was her 2-year-old son Charles Romauld. 17 years later in the Buenos Aires barrio of Bajo Belgrano, at a café-bar populated with jockeys and others from the nearby Palermo racetrack, the 19-year-old singer Charles Romauld Gardès was introduced as 'El Morocho del Abasto' (Abasto being his home barrio). His style was firmly based on that of the two Italian opera stars Enrique Caruso and Titta Ruffo. In a couple of years Charles Romauld Gardès would become known as Carlos Gardel.

During the years of 1910 and 1911 young Carlos Gardel made two connections that began his long journey to international stardom:

- the first was with Saúl Salinas, a leading talent amongst folk singers, guitarists and composers who also worked with many of the tango stars of the day (such as singer Alfredo Gobbi and bandoneonist Juan Maglio). In 1911 Salinas introduced Gardel to the proprietor of Casa Tagini (music retailer and recently appointed agent for the North American recording company Columbia) and in 1912 Gardel made his first recordings on the Columbia label. Most were his own compositions of folk styles: estilos, cifras, vidalitas, vals, and some simply marked as a song. Gardel was not a singer of tangos, nor aspired to be one, and was described on the record labels simply as an artist of the Teatro Nacional;

- the second connection was with the well-known Uruguayan folk singer and guitarist José Francisco Razzano. The two worked well together singing in unison and occasionally alternating their lines in a 'call and response' fashion, like a co-operating rather than competing payada[55].

Saúl Salinas taught Gardel and Razzan how to vary their duets so that they sang together as two intertwining lines harmonising one with the other. Salinas briefly joined them in a quartet together with Francisco Martino and in August 1913 the newspaper *El Nacional* reported that their provincial airs, estilos, and vidalitas were heard with profound delight. That

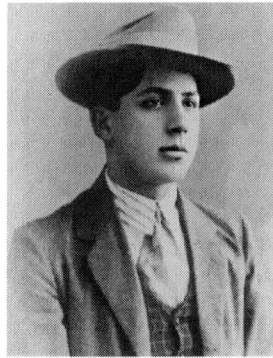

---

[55] payadas were often 'duelling' songs of improvised verse.

innovative approach attracted many followers and the Gardel/Razzano duo was invited to sing on both sides of the Río de la Plata and further afield. On 31 December 1913 Gardel and Razzano were contracted for three months to perform at the high-class cabaret/restaurant Armenonville. Also performing there was tango pianist Roberto Firpo with whom they became friends and frequently toured together. Firpo later recalled that Gardel and Razzano used to drive him crazy with their pranks, jokes, and general indiscipline. In any event Gardel's fame accelerated and he and Razzano were playing almost non-stop in city centre theatres, the seaside resort of Mar del Plata, and across the provinces and neighbouring countries. Some decades later Razzano remembered, very specifically on 17 August 1915, that they were both on the ship *SS Infanta Isobel* heading for Brazil and on board, returning from his performances in Buenos Aires, was Gardel's idol the recording star Enrique Caruso who praised Gardel's singing.

In December 1915 Gardel's career and life nearly ended abruptly with his attempted murder. Gardel had developed a relationship with a woman. Jeanne (sometimes Giovanna) Ritana was an influential woman in the nightclub and night entertainment scene and as a result Gardel had many eyes upon him, few of them benevolent. On 10 December 1915 he was confronted by Ritana's business partner and lover, Amadeo Garesio, and threats were made followed by a scuffle. Some say that Gardel fled by car and was pursued, others say that he stood his ground[56]. Whatever the sequence of events the confrontation ended when one of Garesio's hired men pulled out a gun and fired. Carlos Gardel fell to the

---

[56] other details have varied in the telling, some say it was 11 December because it neatly falls on Gardel's birthday, others that it was Gardel's friend Elias Alippi who was attacked

ground. The following day the newspaper *La Nación* reported that a man had been taken to a hospital with a serious gunshot wound. Years later the examining surgeon explained that the bullet had punctured Gardel's lung and lodged in his chest. Due to the complexity of operating safely the surgeon decided to leave the bullet in place and make the necessary repairs around it. In the newspaper *La Razón* on 14 February 1916 Gardel said that although the bullet was still inside him he could not feel it and it did not trouble him.

The man behind the whole shooting drama, the nightclub owner and part-time gangster Amadeo Garesio became (in the following decade) a pioneer promoter of tango. In 1924 he took ownership of the nightclub El Chantecler attracting the rich, famous, and infamous. That year he hired the new sextet headed by Julio De Caro. In 1925, in his role of agent for performing artists, Garesio secured the contract that sent Francisco Canaro to Paris thereby contributing to another phase of tango frenzy in Parisian high society. And in the early 1930s he invited a new orchestra with a much simpler, rhythmic and energetic style to El Chantecler - led by Juan D'Arienzo. In summary, the little known Amadeo Garesio managed in a couple of decades to both promote pioneering tango stars and nearly kill one.

In April 1917 Gardel and Razzano were contracted by Max Glücksmann's Odeon and recorded 25 tracks of their usual mix of national creole songs. The record advertisements described them as modest, good, patriotic and having the souls of artists and visions of poets. Gardel also recorded *El Noche Triste* that was neither the first performance of this sung tango nor the launch of its fame but in retrospect it marked the blending of tango with rich vocal intonation, as opposed to the earlier, harsher vocal styles of Villoldo, Gobbi, and payadors Ezeiza and Cazón[57].

At that time Roberto Firpo's quintet was also in the Odeon studio and was recording an instrumental and tango version of the well-known estilo (a folk genre) *El Moro*. The story told is that Gardel and Razzano entered unannounced, as one of many pranks they played on Firpo, and sang the chorus. The recording does not capture the undoubted confusion that ensued and so presumably the outcome was considered worthy of a more orderly re-take. Whilst the quintet played, Gardel and Razzano sang only the chorus (twice) thereby unintentionally creating the first recording with the tango estribillista (singer of the refrain)[58]. Yet despite Gardel and Razzano being popular artists their names did not appear on the record label - this was a Firpo record for the dance market.

Despite the wound to his lung and extra piece of metal in his chest Carlos Gardel went on to improve his powerful delivery of tango songs for another 20 years until his sudden and dramatic death in 1935[59].

---

[57] see *Get To Know the Tango Pioneers Origins to 1909*

[58] see more on the estribillista in *Get To Know the Tango Pioneers 1920 to 1935*

[59] Gardel was on board an aeroplane awaiting take off when another aircraft crashed in to it. He and many of his entourage died in the resulting blaze

Arturo Mathón

Arturo Mathón was a composer, singer and guitarist of national aires (estilos, cifras, gatos, and tangos). He is sometimes described as a payador but his appreciated skill was not his improvised verse but his lyrics, his melody, and his voice. People listened attentively. He is little known today but he was a bridge between folk and tango. He preceded the recordings of Francisco Bianco (above) and was the first to record with an orquesta típica although his voice did not maintain a tight rhythm for dancing like Bianco's. You can listen to several of his tango recordings on YouTube and the DAHR website, particulary *El apache argentino* and *El cachafaz*.

- in 1912 he made 24 recordings (on the Columbia label at the Casa Tagini) including 6 tangos. Mathón sang and played guitar and the other artist, Francisco Raya, accompanied him on the bandoneón. On 28 March 1913 the Casa Tagini advertised its Repertoire Criollo in the magazine Fray Mocho where it described Raya's instrument as the 'bandoleón' and both of them as 'Artistas del Teatro Nacional';

- in 1914, again on the Columbia label, Mathón recorded 30 tracks including 10 tangos accompanied by an orquesta típica of unknown musicians, often mistakenly identified as that of Juan Maglio. The majority of recordings were Mathón's own compositions. Unfortunately none of his compositions nor lyrics are heard today because they were were not re-recorded in the later era of improved recording technology. That absence of recordings does not diminish his importance as an influential tango pioneer.

Lola Membrives

Lola Membrives was born in 1888 in Buenos Aires but first made
her name as an actress, singer, and recording artist in Spain[60]. She
returned to Buenos Aires and as tangos became more popular in
theatre productions so too did the actresses who sang them. In
1909 she had recorded the ubiquitous tango *La morocha*
accompanied on piano by the renowned playwright, theatre
impresario, and tango composer Antonio Reynoso. Her voice is
not easy on today's ears but she was clearly popular and delivered
tangos in the fashionable style of the Spanish copla and tonadilla[61].

In 1916 Max Glücksmann of Casa Lepage not only recorded and
promoted her as one of his few top stars but also gave Lola her own
record label 'Disco Lola Membrives' bearing her photograph. On
19 November 1916 Membrives wrote to Max Glücksmann
thanking him because she said that it was only Odeon that could
manage to achieve an exact recording of her voice. In 1917 she
recorded the tango *Cara sucia*. In 1919 she recorded it again
supported by the orchestra of Francisco Canaro and in 1924 she
recorded the tango *La Milonguita* supported by the orchestra of
Roberto Firpo.

In 1924 Lola's photograph was included in an advertisement for
Max Glücksmann's Nacional Odeon and she was in good
company, the only other photographs were of the superstars

---

[60] she recorded in Barcelona in 1903

[61] despite breaking in to the tango market she remained known as a singer in the
Spanish-style. In the magazine *La Nota* (18 September 1916) she was described as a
star of the copla and in the magazine *PBT* (4 August 1917) undeservedly as the
creator of the tonadilla

Roberto Firpo, Carlos Gardel and José Razzano. Her advertised record was a tango for the dance floor, *La chismosa*, another of many compositions that remain unknown to today's tango fans.

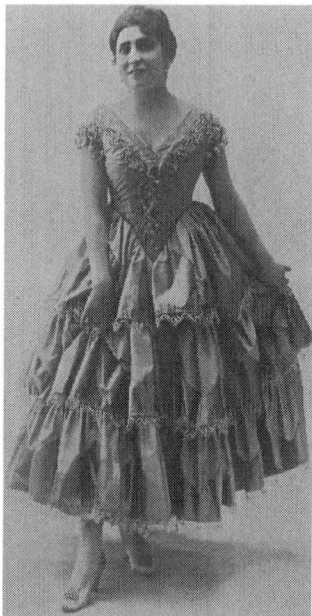

3. The Pianists

Bardi, Cobían, De Bassi, Delfino, Di Sarli, Ferrer, Firpo,
Geroni Flores, Lomuto, Martínez, Rizutti

Agustín Bardi

Agustín Bardi is best known today firstly as a composer of tangos and then as a pianist but at the age 23 years old (in 1908) he was doing neither. He was beginning to play the violin but he had no intention of doing so in order to make a living because for him the late night life of a musician with uncertain income held little appeal. He had, and would continue to hold, a regular office job in the haulage industry. However his passion was tango music and in the evenings, when he could, he did join his musician friends. In 1912 he was playing violin in the tango trio of bandoneonist Genaro Espósito with guitarist Félix Camarano. In the same year he was at the Café Argentino playing piano in the tango quartet of bandoneonist Graciano De Leone alongside violinist David 'Tito' Roccatagliata and flautist Carlos Hernani Macchi. It was also from that year that he started to compose.

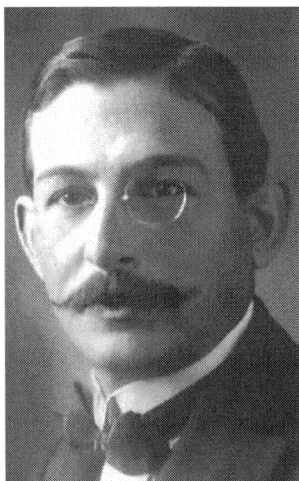

The winter of 1918 was an extraordinary one as residents were amazed to witness snow falling on the city. It remains one of those years that is still remembered and remarked upon today, when the subject of snow and Buenos Aires arises. Agustín composed his latest, as yet unnamed, tango and when he arrived at a meeting to share it with friends, bursting through the door he exclaimed 'What a night!'. They helped him with what they considered to be an obvious title: *Qué noche*. It was recorded by Osvaldo Fresedo performing as the Orquesta Típica Select in New York (1920), by both Julio De Caro and Roberto Firpo (1930), but is best known today by the version of Juan D'Arienzo (1937).

Bardi continued to be an admired tango pianist and composer through the following two decades until 1941 when he died aged 56. He was honoured by Osvaldo Pugliese's tribute tango *Adiós Bardi* (1944) that was also recorded by Juan D'Arienzo (1967) and Aníbal Troilo (1970). Tango pianist Horacio Salgan composed his own tribute *Don Agustín Bardi* and recorded it in 1950 followed by the version by Osvaldo Pugliese (1961).

Bardi's other tango compositions include the still popular:

COMPOSITION	BEST KNOWN RECORDED VERSIONS
Lorenzo	Juan D'Arienzo (1936), Francisco Canaro (1938)
Gallo ciego	Juan D'Arienzo (1937), Ricardo Tanturi (1938), Osvaldo Pugliese (1959)
CTV	Orquesta Típica Victor (1932), Aníbal Troilo (1942),
Nunca tuvo novio	Orquesta Típica Victor (1930), Pedro Laurenz (1943)
La racha	Lucio Demare (1938), Carlos Di Sarli (1947)

El buey solo	Francisco Canaro (1935), Ricardo Tanturi (1941)
Se le llevaron	Orquesta Típica Victor (1937), Francisco Canaro (1937)
Tinta verde	Juan D'Arienzo (1935), Aníbal Troilo (1938), Carlos Di Sarli (1945, 1954)
Tierrita	Edgardo Donato (1934), Ricardo Tanturi (1937), Juan D'Arienzo (1941)

Juan Carlos Cobián

María Silvana Coria, wife of Manuel Cobián, gave birth to Juan Carlos in 1896 in the town of Pigüé, north of Bahia Blanca. The family home had a piano and several of his siblings could play. Juan Carlos took a particularly keen interest and was formally schooled at the famous Williams Conservatory in Bahia Blanca[62]. In 1913, aged 18, Juan Carlos arrived in central Buenos Aires. There he played at the silent cinema *Las Familias* (in the present day Barrio Norte) where during the intervals he performed the tango *El Caburé*, the 1911 hit composed by Arturo De Bassi. The cinema manager was impressed and told his friend who came along to hear for himself and was equally excited. That friend happened to be bandoneonist Eduardo Arolas who recommended to Cobían that he should hang around at the Bar Iglesias on Calle Corrientes where all the regulars were tango musicians. It was

---

[62] where some years later another tango pioneer, Carlos Di Sarli, would study

there that Cobían watched and met the resident quartet of bandoneonist Genaro Espósito, violinists Ernesto Zambonini and Alcides Palavecino, and pianist Roberto Firpo.

In 1914 Roberto Firpo won a competition to form the resident tango group for the Armenonville cabaret that left the Espósito quartet without a pianist. Arolas recommended Espósito to go to *Las Familias* cinema to check out the young Cobían in action. Almost immediately Cobían found himself in a makeshift nightclub in the backyard of a bakery playing alongside the pleasant but musically illiterate Genaro Espósito and the often drunk and disagreeable Ernesto Zambonini. Opposite the bakery was the famous Teatro Politeama where two decades later, in February 1937, Cobían would be inside directing the carnival orchestra consisting of the outstanding bandoneonists Aníbal Troilo and Ciriaco Ortiz, violinists Cayetano Puglisi and Hugo Baralis, and pianist Orlando Goñi. However returning to the bakery backyard, the refined Juan Carlos Cobían knew that the venue was not his natural environment nor were Espósito and Zambonini his kind of musicians nor company. He soon found a more pleasing position providing the music at the dance studio of the famous Juan Carlos Herrera, who we met in the *Dancers* section above.

Despite his earlier discomfort with the venues and musicians of the arrabal, Cobían was still drawn to the earthiness of the music and was soon touring with bandoneonist Ricardo 'Mochila' Gonzalez and violinist Julio Doutry. He should not have been surprised to have found the tour to have been as unpleasant as his experiences with Espósito and so he parted ways and found an improved opportunity to work with bandoneonist Vicente Greco and violinist Ricardo Gaudenzio. The difference was that, following Greco's newly found fame as the first recorded orquesta típica criolla, his venues were in luxury hotels and the private residences of high society. That was Cobían's natural habitat. Over the next couple of years Cobían played in hotels, restaurants, cabarets, and grand houses in two trios: with guitarist-turned-bandoneonist Graciano De Leone and violinist Juan Pedro Castillo[63]; and another with Eduardo Arolas and violinist David 'Tito' Roccatagliata. In 1917 Arolas left the latter trio and so Cobían and Roccagliata needed to find a replacement bandoneonist. The 20-year-old Osvaldo Fresedo matched perfectly Cobian's idea of a tango musician - educated and refined. Roccatagliata less so as, after several years of close working with Arolas, he was a committed consumer of strong alcohol. Nevertheless the three of them formed a team completely aligned in their style of tango and became good personal friends living together in a small apartment. Inspired by the appreciative reactions of their audiences Cobían continued to develop a tango structure with a broader base of 4x8 rather than the traditional 2x4. That allowed him to build in more interplay of counter melodies and decorative bass runs with his left hand that had not hitherto been heard but would soon become known as the distinctive and innovative Cobían style. His dexterity and lightness of touch earned him the nicknames of the 'Chopin of Tango'[64] and the 'Aristocrat of Tango'.

At the end of 1918 the successful and much loved trio of Cobían, Fresedo, and Roccatgliatta went their separate ways. In 1920 Cobían joined the veteran bandoneonist Arturo Bernstein for a well-paid contract at the prestigious Hotel Victoria in Córdoba. Later back in Buenos Aires, Cobían formed the Orquesta Goubián,

---

[63] known at the time as one of the best pizzicato players in the tango business (pizzicato being the technique of plucking the violin strings)
[64] one should not try to find musical similarities between Chopin and Cobían, the sobriquet was simply to pay respect to Cobían

apparently deliberately misspelling his surname to avoid his obligatory national service in the armed forces. Unsurprisingly, he was eventually caught and punished with a short spell in a military prison, where he composed a tango based on his punitive meal of bread and water: *Pan y aqua*[65].

Arturo De Bassi

By 1910 Arturo De Bassi, still only 20 years old, had already proved himself as a successful tango composer and now was directing the Banda Ítalo-Argentina and making a couple of recordings on the Odeon label including his own tango composition *El incendio*. De Bassi composed another tango *El caburé* that remains popular today. It is often mistakenly dated as being premiered in 1909 in the play *El caburé* for which De Bassi had provided the music. However he did not compose it until 1911 and named it *El caburé* in order to build on the commercial success of the earlier play. It was a shrewd move as in February 1913 the magazine *PBT* reported the accumulated sale of 100,000 copies of the *El caburé* sheet music over the previous few months. It continued as a long-lasting success and when reviewing his career in 1937 De Bassi considered it to be his personal favourite. *El caburé* was almost immediately recorded by the

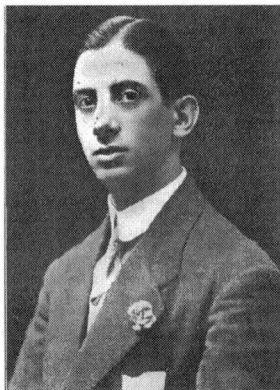

El maestro Arturo de Bassi, director de la gran banda-orquesta que actuará en el teatro Casino, en los bailes de máscaras de los días 4, 5, 6, 7, 11 y 12 de marzo.

---

[65] best known by the recording of Ángel D'Agostino and singer Ángel Vargas (1945)

Rondalla del Gaucho Relámpago and by Juan Maglio but we know it best today through the versions of, amongst others: Roberto Firpo (1927), Adolfo Carabelli (1932), Francisco Canaro (1936), Juan D'Arienzo (1937), and Carlos Di Sarli (1946 and 1951). The film *La Cabalgata del Circo,* although released in 1945, included a scene of the tango *El caburé* in the style setting of about 1911. The singers were tango stars Hugo del Carril and Libertad Lamarque and the music was depicted as being provided by a street organito.

In late 1912 Alfredo Améndola had set up his Atlanta recording facilities in Buenos Aires and he asked Arturo De Bassi to form and direct two 'house bands': the Rondalla Atlanta (stringed instruments) and the Banda Atlanta (brass and woodwind instruments). Amongst the 170 recordings (in 1912/1913) were a couple of dozen tangos most of which are, regrettabaly, no longer familiar to us today.

Between the 5th and 12th March 1916 De Bassi was directing the orchestra at the Teatro Casino for the carnival week. In the advertisements the venue was described as the most modern and luxurious carnival event ever to be held. The Casino had a sliding roof open to the outside air with 150 fans to help the fresh air to circulate, more than 20 electric lights to produce daylight in the evenings, and everywhere was beautifully decorated. De Bassi's orchestra was to be the largest and the most highly talented ever assembled and would play 'plentiful and beautiful tangos'. The carnival event would also include competitions for the best couples dancing tangos. In the absence of film or recordings we are left to imagine the scene and the sound of the orchestra playing the most popular tangos of the day, the excitable partygoers, and the dancers (some more earnestly competitive than others). And then we should pause to remember that this tango extravaganza was in 1916, decades before the supposed 'Golden Age' of the 1940s.

In addition to *El caburé* Arturo's other tango compositions still heard today include:

COMPOSITION	BEST KNOWN RECORDED VERSIONS
El incendio	Rodolfo Biagi (1938), Carlos Di Sarli (1940 and 1951), Alfredo Gobbi Junior (1948)
La catrera	Juan D'Arienzo (1938, 1949, 1955, 1963), Alfredo Gobbi Junior (1951), Héctor Varela (1957)
Don Pacifico	Juan D'Arienzo (1939, 1949, and 1954)
Mano blanca	Angel D'Agostino (1944)
Manón	Alfredo Carabelli (1932), Osvaldo Fresedo (1942), Osvaldo Pugliese (1969)

In the following decades Arturo De Bassi successfully established his career in the world of theatre productions. On 17 June 1950 he heard his composition *El incendio* on the radio performed by the orchestra of Carlos Di Sarli. Pleased with the rendition he telephoned his congratulations to Di Sarli thanking him for choosing to play his tango. Later that same day Arturo suffered a heart attack and passed away, aged 60.

Enrique Delfino

Enrique Pedro Delfino was born in Buenos Aires in 1895. His parents ran the confiteria at the Teatro Politeama, the leading theatre of musical productions and the location of the largest carnival events. Enrique was therefore never far away from the world of musical entertainment. Additionally his parents ensured he received the best professional music education including classical training in Turin, Italy. By the age of 17 Enrique Delfino was a virtuoso pianist and travelled to Montevideo to perform not refined recitals at concert halls but at the pianos of café-bars and silent cinemas. Whilst there he also started to compose tangos. His first composition, in 1912, became an outstanding success and versions of it are still regularly heard at today's milongas around the world: *Re fa si*. Unfortunately for him he did not receive the financial rewards he deserved as he was pleased enough (at the time) to sell the rights to a music publisher for only 35 pesos. It was recorded in 1917 by Roberto Firpo but is best known today by the versions of Orquesta Típica Victor (1927), Juan D'Arienzo (1935), Rodolfo Biagi (1940), and Carlos Di Sarli (1953). In 1914 he composed the tango *Bélgica* (moved by the accounts coming from Europe at the start of the World War). The composition had a different feel to the contemporary tangos and many now say that it marked the start of

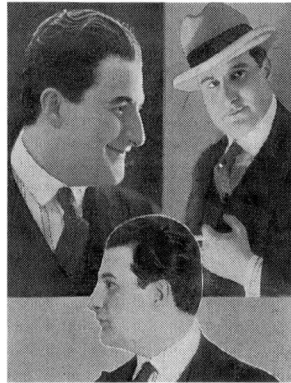

the 'tango romanza' genre[66] - a style of composition that was followed by bandoneonist Osvaldo Fresedo, pianist Juan Carlos Cobían, violinist Julio De Caro and others. Fresedo recorded *Bélgica* as a bandoneón solo in 1920 (whilst he was with Delfino in the USA) but it is best known today by the much more rhythmic, syncopated, and not at all 'romanza' 1942 recording by Rodolfo Biagi.

On 10 May 1917, in Buenos Aires, Delfino entered the temporary recording room at the premises of retailer Pratt & Co and recorded (on the Victor label) 4 piano solos including his own composition *Sans Souci*, that is best known today by the recordings by Juan D'Arienzo (1942) and Miguel Caló (1944). I do not know what he was doing on the 12 May but he was supposed to have been recording another two tracks. The sound engineer noted in the ledger 'Was to come back Saturday for two make overs   - disappointed us!'.

In 1918 Delfino was again in Montevideo, accompanying the bandoneonist José Quevado and violinist Edgardo Donato. In 1920 he would head off on an adventure to the Victor recording studios in the USA to form the Orquesta Típica Select together with bandoneonist Osvaldo Fresedo and violinist David Roccatagliata[67].

---

[66] There is no technical definition but indicates a musically lyrical style. One could say more sophisticated than tango for the dance floor (known as tango milonga)
[67] see *Get To Know the Tango Pioneers 1920 to 1935*

Carlos Di Sarli

Carlos Di Sarli is known today as a tango pianist, composer, and orchestra leader and his recordings (from 1928 to 1958) are still heard and adored at nearly every tango social dance event around the world.

He was born in 1903 in the city of Bahía Blanca, some 630 kilometres south of Buenos Aires, and raised in a musical family. His mother Serafina Russomano came from a musically talented family in Montevideo, Uruguay and her siblings were pianists and singers[68]. Serafina met a recently arrived Italian immigrant and widower with three children, Miguel Di Sarli, who shared her love of music. They married and had four of their own children. Miguel Di Sarli became a teacher at the Montevideo School of Arts and Crafts and made friends with music teacher José Spátola. In 1923 the Spátola family would play a pivotal role in the career of Miguel's as yet unborn son Carlos Di Sarli. Life in Montevideo was reasonably happy and stable until Miguel became active in the divisive politics of the Uruguayan Blancos fighting against the Colorados. Following a defeat in 1897 many of the Blanco supporters feared for their safety and emigrated to Argentina. Miguel and his family were amongst them and they eventually settled in the town of Bahía Blanca where Miguel opened a gun shop. The Di Sarlis added to their already extensive family with the birth of two more sons, Cayetano in 1903 (who would later rename himself Carlos) followed shortly by Roque. All of the Di Sarli children were brought up with music in the home: Nicolas became a baritone singer like his uncle Tito; Domingo became a teacher at

---

[68] her older brother Tito became a renowned tenor

the local music academy; and Cayetano (Carlos) and Roque became pianists.

In 1916, aged just 13 years, Cayetano Di Sarli ran away from home to join a female travelling theatre group touring the provinces around Bahía Blanca. His anxious parents, having retrieved him, appeased his quest for adventure by sending him to a family friend in La Pampa who owned a confiteria and silent cinema. There Cayetano (soon to rename himself Carlos) spent the next couple of years at the piano entertaining audiences and developing his tango technique.

In 1919 Carlos Di Sarli returned from La Pampa to his parents' home in Bahía Blanca and secured work as the resident pianist at the local Café Paulista. It was an unusual arrangement for a pianist as the café did not have a piano. Carlos had to push his own piano from home through the streets to the café where he and it stayed for nearly three years. In that same year Di Sarli lost his eye from a gunshot in his father's armoury. The circumstances told by the Di Sarli family over the years have varied from being accidentally shot by an intruder, by a careless employee, and deliberately by Carlos himself in a bout of lovesick depression. Whilst the true reason remains a mystery Carlos Di Sarli became distinctive not only for his excellent tango music but also for his permanent wearing of dark glasses.

In 1923 Di Sarli moved to Buenos Aires but success did not come easily and for a variety of reasons he attracted the resentment of many in the music business.

Celestino Ferrer

Celestino Ferrer was a pianist and orchestra leader who recorded prolifically. Although the discs were destined for and sold in Argentina they were all recorded abroad. Between 1913 and 1919 he recorded with Pathé in France and with both Victor and Columbia in the USA.

Celestino Ferrer was born in 1885 in Buenos Aires and became a pianist playing tangos in café-bars during the first decade of the 1900s. He came to the wider public's attention in April 1913 thanks to an article in the Buenos Aires magazine *Sherlock Holmes*. Although the article was primarily about the dance studio of Casimiro Ain in the basement of a café, the journalist expanded his interest to the wonders of the café's tango quartet. The article included the musicians in one of the photographs (below, showing Celestino Ferrer seated at the piano, Vicente Loduca to the left, Eduardo Monelos standing, and to the far right was José Sentio).

Two months later Ferrer, Loduca and Monelos were performing on stage in Paris together with the dancer Casimiro Ain and his partner. The trio of musicians made nearly 60 recordings of tangos and vals on the Pathé label, marketed variously as the Rondalla Criollo Ferrer, Orquesta Típica Loduca, and Orquesta Típica Monelos. The names did not indicate any shift in leadership of the trio nor any change in their choice of recordings or style but was simply a marketing device to cynically increase the apparent number of different artists in the Pathé catalogue. The records went on sale in Buenos Aires from October 1913 and included many of the favourite compositions of the day, some of which are still familiar (due to recordings by later orchestras): *Una Noche de garufa, De pura cepa, Rodríguez Peña, Un copetín, Independencia, Argañaraz, Viento en popa, El tamango, El caburé, El irresistible, Siete palabras, Sentimiento criollo, Mate amargo,* and the valses *Francia, Pabellón de las Rosas, Amor y Primavera, Lagrimas y sonrisas.*

Later that year Ferrer, Loduca, and Monelos sailed to New York and on 7 January 1914 were in the Victor laboratories at Camden, New Jersey recording as the Orquesta Típíca Argentina Loduca. After the recording contract had concluded Vicente Loduca then headed south to Brazil[69] and Eduardo Monelos returned home to Argentina. Ferrer decided to extend his international adventures and returned to Europe but he needed replacement musicians. He sent for his former colleague from Buenos Aires the violinist José Sentio and bandoneonist Güerino Filipotto. By July 1914 Ferrer, Filipotto, and Sentio were performing in central Paris venues, together with the dancer Casimiro Ain. Within a month Germany

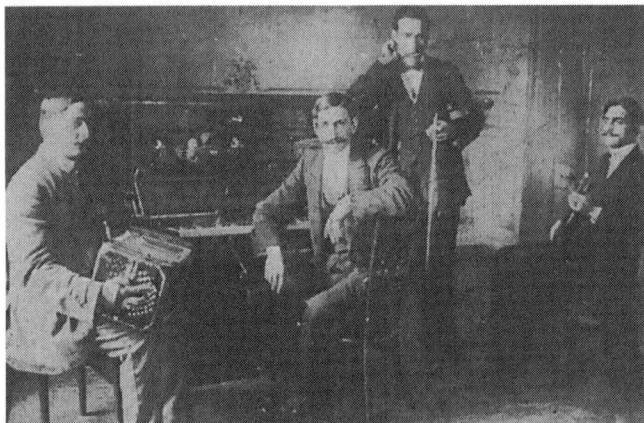

---

[69] there are unconfirmed reports of him being contracted to perform there as a professional magician.

declared war on France, the British Empire declared war on Germany and everything changed.

In April 1915 Ferrer was back in the USA and recording (at the Victor Talking Machine Company) as both the Orquesta Argentina de Ferrer and the Orquesta Típica Argentino Celestino. They were both quintets and both with local session artists that included an accordionist (in the absence of any North American bandoneón players). Bandoneonist Güerino Filipotto was not mentioned as a musician in the Victor ledgers until November 1915. Between 1915 and 1919 Ferrer recorded as many as 125 tracks that included tangos that are well-known today (due to later orchestras):

TITLE	BEST KNOWN RECORDED VERSIONS
Didi	Roberto Firpo (1937), Rodolfo Biagi (1941), Ricardo Tanturi (1941), Carlos Di Sarli (1947 and 1951)
Una noche de garufa	Ricardo Tanturi (1941)
La payanca	Orquesta Típica Victor (1926), Juan D'Arienzo (1936), Roberto Firpo (1946)
El estagiario	Edgardo Donato (1938), Carlos Di Sarli (1941)
El Pollo Ricardo	Francisco Canaro (1938), Carlos Di Sarli (1940, 1946, and 1951)

By the end of 1919 Ferrer and Filipotto had moved from Victor to the Columbia label and recorded a couple of dozen tracks as the Orquesta Ferrer Filipotto. Most of them can be heard on the DAHR[70] website and whilst many titles are no longer familiar to us

---

[70] Discography of American Historical Recordings

today there are some that we do recognise (again, due to the recordings of later orchestras):

TITLE	BEST KNOWN RECORDED VERSIONS
Don Esteban	Juan D'Arienzo (1936), Francisco Canaro (1938)
Muñequita	Francisco Lomuto (1927, 1931, 1940), Ángel D'Agostino (1944)
Mano brava	Francisco Canaro (1940, 1956)
Un lamento	Carlos Di Sarli (1929, 1944, 1953), Ángel D'Agostino (1942)
Pampa	Francisco Canaro (1938), Juan D'Arienzo (1939, 1951)

On 1 November 1919 Victor advertised the recordings of the Orquesta Típica Argentina de Ferrer although each record label

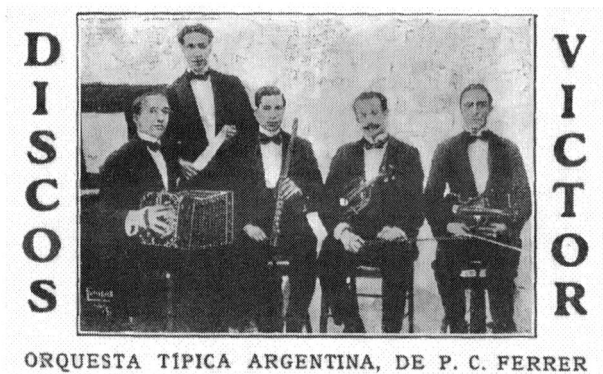

ORQUESTA TÍPICA ARGENTINA, DE P. C. FERRER

was individually marked Orquesta Típica Celestino – it is of course the same person and the same quintet. The photograph shows Ferrer standing by his piano, the bandoneónist Güerino Filipotto, and two North American session violinists and a flautist. Amongst their recordings were two piano solos by Ferrer and a tango *Co-Co*, that is unknown today but the main interest to us is that it was composed by Antonio Tanturi, a tango orchestra leader long before his younger, better known, brother Ricardo[71]. Their other recorded tangos included those composed by the pioneers Enrique Delfino, Augusto Berto, Juan Maglio, and Alberico Spátola.

Ferrer and Filipotto then returned once again to Paris and became a key part of the next tango craze. In the early 1920s the Orchestre Argentin Ferrer Filipotto played at the cabaret Garron and at the opening dance night at the Theatre Apollo. At the same time they joined forces with the recently arrived Argentinian musicians Manual Pizarro and Genaro Espósito. By 1926 Filipotto was leading his own orchestra and recorded at the Savoy Hotel in London as the Filipotto and (Francisco) Ariotto Tango Band. Celestino Ferrer settled in Europe and passed away in Germany in 1958, aged 72.

---

[71] Ricardo Tanturi's recordings from 1940 to 1950 are still regularly heard at milongas around the world

Roberto Firpo

This is the decade (1910 to 1919) in which Roberto Firpo established himself as the leading tango performer, particularly on recordings.

Recordings

On 16 April 1911 Max Birckhahn, a recording engineer, sailed on the *Cap Vilano* from Hamburg to Buenos Aires with portable equipment in order to record local artists and to transport the masters back to Germany for the production of records on the labels of ERA, BEKA, Odeon, Parlophone and others[72]. The ERA Buenos Aires agent was Carlos Nasca who, as well as recording himself as the Rondalla del Gaucho Relámpago, invited Roberto Firpo to make his first recordings: piano solos and duets with a violinist. In 1912 Juan Tagini had also arranged for German engineers to visit and record on the Columbia label at his retail premises of Casa Tagini. Amongst the artists was Firpo as the pianist in the Genaro Espósito orquesta típica (actually a trio). In 1913 yet another Buenos Aires businessman, Alfredo Améndola, had made similar arrangements with Germany to record at his premises and produce records on the Atlanta label. There Firpo

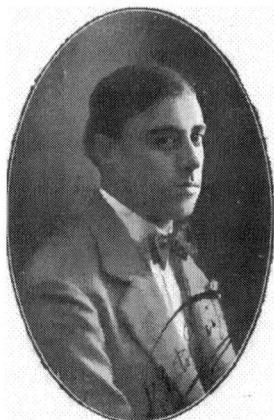

ROBERTO FIRPO

---

[72] many individual companies/trading names/labels had been absorbed within the Carl Lindstrom AG multi-national company in which staff and resources were shared.

recorded at least 14 tracks: his own composition *Sentimiento criollo*, Rosendo Mendizábal's *Viento en popa*, and Manuel Campoamor's *El entrerriano* all of which are still familiar tango compositions today. Firpo's name was also put to about 24 recordings on the ERA label although he did not feature in them. The labels specifically identify an orquesta típica 'directed by Roberto Firpo'. The instruments included a guitar but no piano and so Firpo's input was as musical arranger/director and perhaps more importantly as a marketing device - his name carried a value far beyond his musical input. There are two possible reasons to explain why he did not play the piano on the ERA recordings:

- technical. The capabilities of the portable recording equipment used and/or the conditions of the room meant that the piano could not be captured in balance with the other instruments;
- legal. Firpo had just contracted himself as a performing artist exclusively to Max Glücksmann's Odeon.

In 1914 Firpo was only one of several tango dance orchestras recording on Odeon: others included the orquestas típicas of Eduardo Arolas, Domingo Biggeri, El Rusito (being Antonio Gutman), Rodríguez (directed by José Pécora), and Unión. However from 1915 to 1922 he was the only one. Somehow he had secured a contract that held for 7 years stating that he was to be the only tango orquesta típica to record with Odeon[73]. All of the regular advertisements posted by Max Glücksmann's Odeon were dominated by photographs of Roberto Firpo together with listings of his recordings and compositions. To the general public the words 'tango' and 'Firpo' were synonymous. In 1914 the Orquesta

---

[73] in 1923 Francisco Canaro, Juan Maglio, and Francisco Lomuto managed to squeeze their way in to Odeon, followed in 1926 by Osvaldo Fresedo.

Criolla Firpo (that was a quartet with violinist David Roccatagliata, bandoneonist Juan Deamboggio, and flautist Alejandro Michetti) recorded at least 50 tracks, the vast majority being tangos and his own compositions, and included 5 piano solos including *El amanecer, Marejada,* and *Argañaraz.* It is interesting to listen to the latter and compare it with his quartet's version and of course the more familiar later versions by Ricardo Tanturi (1940), Ángel D'Agostino (1952), and Juan D'Arienzo (1966).

On 19 March 1914 Roberto Firpo wrote to Max Glücksmann

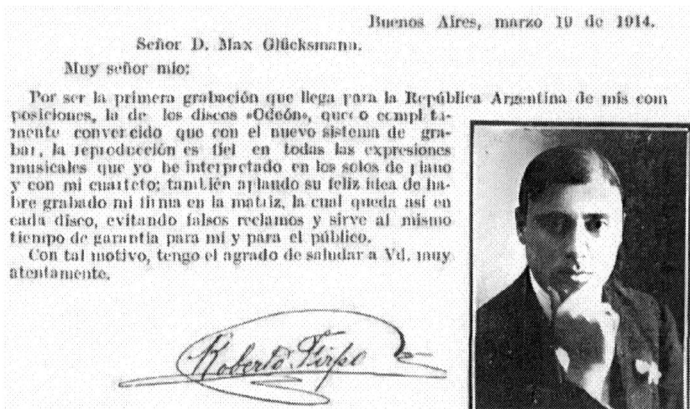

praising him for the quality of the Odeon recordings and the innovative idea of including his signature on each label thereby assuring the listener that the recording was authentic[74]. On 27 March Glücksmann listed the latest recordings by Roberto Firpo of his own compositions: 16 tangos including *De pura cepa, Sentimiento criollo, Argañaraz, Alma de bohemio.* It also included 5 double-sided records of Firpo's piano solos (including one that had on the other side an Eduardo Arolas solo on the 'mandonión', a bizarre mis-

---

[74] it was not so innovative, see *Recordings* above

spelling of bandoneón). Firpo was also employed to accompany other, non-tango, artists presumably because Firpo's name added another reason for the public to buy the record. On 11 November 1916 the Firpo orchestra supported the payador Francisco Bianco singing a vals and estilo and in July 1917 Firpo accompanied the national creole singer and guitarist Saul Salinas.

In 1916 Firpo recorded at least 80 tracks many of which are still familiar compositions today, for example:

- *Alma de bohemio, El amanecer, Didi,* and *El apronte* (composed by Firpo);
- *Germaine* and *Entre dos fuegos* (composed by Alberto Buchardo); and
- *El flete* (composed by Vicente Greco).

Firpo had already recorded and released several of these tangos in the previous years of 1914 and 1915 but there does not appear to have been any decline in interest for the same tangos by the same musicians year after year. That is in part explained by the general acceptance that the grooves in discs eroded after frequent playing and so there was no expectation that a record would be for life.

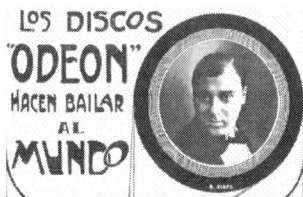

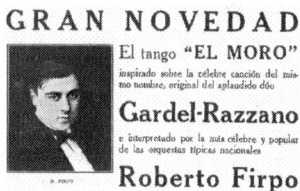

On 27 January 1917 Glücksmann's advertisements declared 'Odeon records make the world dance' – and the only tango dance

records advertised were of course Firpo's. The year was another busy one for Firpo with over 60 recordings. On 22 December Odeon advertised the release of *El Moro* by Firpo saying that it had been inspired by the earlier Gardel and Razzano recording[75]. *El Moro* was a traditional folk song that Firpo had arranged as a tango, demonstrating to us once again the direct influences of folk songs from the Argentinian countryside on the city's early tangos[76].

To appreciate how prolific Firpo was in the recording laboratory it is revealing to look at a snapshot of the recording output of those that are frequently described as the greats of the Golden Age: D'Arienzo, Di Sarli, Troilo, and Pugliese:

- D'Arienzo (over the course of 1935 - 1939) averaged 22 recordings per year;
- Di Sarli (1940 - 1945) averaged 24;
- Troilo (1941 - 1945) averaged 26; and
- Pugliese (1943 - 1952) averaged 28.

Whereas over the course of 1914 to 1919 Firpo averaged 52 recordings per year. The repeated accolade of the Golden Age creates the myth that tango was slowly evolving until it reached its peak interest during the late 1930s to 1950s. The effect is to distort the history of tango and to diminish earlier, equally exciting, golden ages.

Firpo's total recordings during his entire career number about 3000 and yet very few are heard at today's milongas. The reasons are severalfold:

---

[75] see *Singers/Gardel* above
[76] see *Get To Know the Tango Pioneers Origins to 1909*

- most were recorded in the acoustic era and so are of relatively low reproduction sound quality for today's dancers;
- his electric recordings from the late 1920s to early 1930s currently have limited commercial availability and tend to be played as 'specials'[77]; and finally,
- the better quality and more widely available quartet/quintet recordings (late 1930s/1940s) have a different sound to the orquesta típica of the same era and today tend to divide dancers' opinions.

Performances

Although a prolific recording artist Firpo did not limit himself to the Odeon premises. He was constantly performing both as a solo artist and with others. In 1913 he was the pianist in the trio led by Genaro Espósito that had been asked to audition for the position of resident band at the newly opened Cabaret Armenonville. The management selected Roberto Firpo only and asked him to form his own quartet. We can only assume that they had seen something more refined, and appropriate for their new venue, in the presentation and playing of Firpo rather than of Genaro Espósito. That was clearly a difficult moment but show business is show business and Firpo recruited another bandoneonist, Eduardo Arolas.

One of the most often told accounts of Firpo's performances was the one in 1916 at the grand Café La Giralda, Montevideo. He was performing with his quintet (bandoneonist Juan 'Bachicha' Deambroggio, violinists David 'Tito' Roccatagliata and Agesilao Ferrazzano, and flautist Alejandro Michetti) and had finished their

---

[77] at time of writing there are pleasing signs of better quality transfers emerging

performance when a group of young students approached their table and presented a partly completed music sheet for a marching tune. They said that their friend 'Becho' Matos Rodríguez had composed it for their forthcoming annual carnival but they thought that it could be improved by adapting it in to a tango. Firpo tried to help, took it away with him, changed it a bit by adding parts of his own compositions that had not been so successful. The quintet then performed it at La Giralda to the delight of young Matos Rodríguez and the assembled customers. On return to Buenos Aires Firpo recorded it as *La Cumparsita* and within a year Juan Maglio also recorded it. However the tune made little impact with the public and was practically forgotten but subsequently (and perhaps surprisingly) became the most widely recognised tango around the world. A multitude of interpretations were recorded by the great tango dance orchestras of the 1930s to 1950s and it has become a tradition for the final tango of social dance events (milongas) to be one of those versions of *La Cumparsita.*

We have already read that during the carnival season of 1917 he was jointly leading the Firpo-Canaro grand orchestra in Rosario and in 1918 providing tango music at the theatre[78]. He was also busy performing most evenings in the Bar Iglesias and moving on after midnight to play at the Cabaret Pigall. In 1917 he was with his quintet at the Palais De Glace in Recoleta when an 18 year old, Julio De Caro, was encouraged up to the stage by his friends. Firpo graciously allowed him to play, Agesliao Ferrazzano lent De Caro his violin, and the rapturous applause cemented De Caro's resolve to dedicate himself to a life of tango music[79].

---

[78] see *Venues/Carnivals/Theatres* above
[79] see Violinists/De Caro below

Composing

Just as Firpo the musician was ubiquitous so too were his tango compositions - if it wasn't him that was playing and recording them then someone else was. Here are the recordings of the Orquesta Típica Celestino Ferrer advertised on 29 January 1916. Identifying the composers to the general public was clearly a significant selling point, an assurance of the best quality tangos, whereas today the most ardent tango fan tends to be unaware of the composers (often incorrectly crediting the recording artist).

Repertorio de Tangos de

R. FIRPO y F. J. LOMUTO

Tocados por el quinteto que dirige el Sr. C. P. FERRER, y que han llamado la atención del público, por su sabor criollo y buen compás

Discos dobles, 25 cm., $ ᵐ/ₙ. 2.50 cada uno

67601	Toda la Vida, tango. / Recordando el Pasado, vals.	Roberto Firpo / Roberto Firpo	67607	Marsiada, tango criollo. / El Apronte, tango.	Roberto Firpo / Roberto Firpo
67602	Una Partida, tango. / Didí, tango.	Roberto Firpo / Roberto Firpo	67608	El Bisturí, tango. / Alma de Bohemio, tango.	Roberto Firpo / Roberto Firpo
67603	El Inquieto, tango. / La Rezongona, tango argentino	F. J. Lomuto / F. J. Lomuto	67609	Noche de Farra, tango. / Curda Completa, tango.	Roberto Firpo / Roberto Firpo
67604	Mi Vida, vals criollo. / Indiecita, tango criollo.	F. J. Lomuto / Roberto Firpo	67610	Sentimiento Criollo, tango. / El Gallito, tango americano.	Roberto Firpo / Roberto Firpo
67605	Los Guevara, tango. / De mi Flor, tango	Roberto Firpo / Roberto Firpo			

Rogamos al público comparen los discos VICTOR, en calidad, precio y ejecución, con sus similares.

VICTOR TALKING MACHINE Co.
CAMDEN, N. Y., E. U. de A.

República Argentina
PRATT & Cía.
108, Calle San Martín, 112 — BUENOS AIRES
Calle Córdoba esquina Maipú — ROSARIO

Carlos Geroni Flores

Alejandro Carlos Vicente Geroni was born in 1895 and at some point he picked up the nickname 'El Negro Flores' and was for evermore known as Geroni Flores or the more formalised title C.V.G. Flores. To clarify some possible confusion, born 18 months later in Buenos Aires was the tango poet Celedonio Flores who also became known as 'El Negro Flores'[80].

The father of Carlos Geroni was an educated and cultured man who frequently travelled to Europe, due to his profession in the leather trade, and in 1906 a friend of his from Portugal visited Buenos Aires. Juan Ramozkla happened to be the director of the Royal Music Academy in Lisbon and offered a place to young Carlos who travelled there later that year, aged 11, completed his studies and returned in 1912 as a professional violinist and pianist.

Just before he had left Buenos Aires young Carlos Geroni in 1905 had already touched the world of tango music by transcribing in to musical notation the bandoneonist Vicente Greco's newly composed tango *El Pibe*. The two remained friends and Greco dedicated his tango *El morochito* 'to my friend Carlos Geroni'.

When Geroni returned to Buenos Aires in 1912 he played some prestigious classical concerts: as lead violinist in the visiting troupe of the Milan opera, and in the Salon La Argentina. In 1912 Enrique Saborido, by then a famous pianist and tango composer (*La morocha, Felicia*), was planning a trip to entertain the high society in Paris and to teach them to dance tango. He invited Geroni to be his pianist. In 1913 they were performing in the homes of the

---

[80] Celedonio makes his appearance in *Get To Know the Tango Pioneers 1920 to 1935*

French President Raymond Poincaré, the Baron de Rothschild, and many of the wealthy Parisian aristocrats. They promoted their version of the 'true' Argentinian tango, teaching and judging competitions, and performing at venues such as the Theatre Royal in Paris and the Savoy Hotel in London. In an interview in 1928 Geroni recalled that their most popular tangos included *El irresistible, Sentimiento criollo,* and *La morocha* that remain firm favourites amongst today's tango fans.

Everything came to a halt with the outbreak of the World War. In 1915 the two made their way to the neutral Netherlands and boarded the *SS Turbantia* to return home to Buenos Aires via England, Brazil, and Uruguay. The journey was not without risk as their ship narrowly escaped a submarine attack off the coast of Lisbon[81]. Once safely home Saborido left his life of tango for the more stable one of a public servant, surfacing again in 1932 as the pianist in a revival group playing old style tangos (known as Guardia Vieja[82]). On the other hand the classically trained Geroni returned as a tango convert. He immediately joined the group of bandoneonist veteran Arturo Bernstein[83] and in 1918 he was in a quintet with violinists Agesilao Ferrazzano and Bernardo Germino and bandoneonists Ricardo Brignolo and Roque Biafore. In 1919 he assembled his own sextet with bandoneonists Luis Petrucelli and Carlos Marcucci, and violinists Emilio Ferrer and Esteban Rovati. In 1922 he secured a contract with Victor and made 24 recordings.

---

[81] the *SS Turbantia* was not so lucky the following year when it was struck by a torpedo in the North sea and sunk

[82] See more about the terms Guardia Vieja and Guardia Nueva in *Get To Know the Tango Pioneers Origens to 1909*

[83] by then aged 33.

Francisco Lomuto

Victor and Rosalia Lomuto created a home filled with music and their children became talented musicians. In 1893 their second child, Francisco Juan, was born and within a couple of decades was at the centre of the new-style tango music scene. Two years after Francisco's birth came the arrival of brother Victor who also grew to become a tango musician (a guitarist turned bandoneonist) and established himself in Paris in the 1920s playing with the orchestras of Eduardo Arolas, Genaro Espósito, and Manuel Pizarro. In 1899 Oscar was born and took a different path to his musical brothers by becoming a journalist, although he did use his creative skills to produce the lyrics for the tango *Nunca más*[84]. In 1906 Victor and Rosalía had another son Enrique who became a pianist and orchestra leader and in 1914 their final child was born - Hector, who became a successful jazz band leader in the 1940s and 1950s.

In 1906 Francisco Lomuto is said to have composed, and published, the music for his first tango *El 606*. He was 13 years old. Two years later he was playing the piano to promote the sales of sheet music and records at a music store in the city centre (Avelino Cabezas where Juan

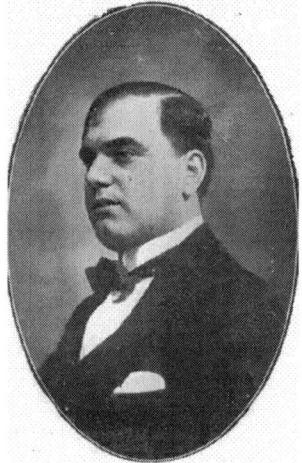

F. J. LOMUTO

D'Arienzo would similarly be working just a few years later). His time there enabled him to focus on the variety of composers' styles,

---

[84] recorded by Francisco Lomuto (1931, 1950)

an exercise that interested him more than performing. Nevertheless he did perform occasionally, for example in 1914 he formed a piano duo with Héctor Quesada; in 1916 he briefly joined a quartet at the Café Monterrey alongside bandoneonist Pedro Maffia; and he played a few sets with the Francico Canaro quintet at the Cabaret Royal. He did have ideas of forming his own orchestra but during the years of this book his fame came from his compositions. The newspapers advertised records of the orchestras of Celestino Ferrer and of Vicente Loduca and identified the composer of the tangos as FJ Lomuto. He was so well regarded that on 12 February 1916 his photograph appeared wearing elegant evening wear and bow tie alongside the other great tango composer Roberto Firpo. His advertised compositions are today little, or not at all, known but did include:

COMPOSITION	BEST KNOWN RECORDED VERSIONS
La rezongona	Francisco Lomuto (1938), Francisco Canaro (1939)
La revoltosa	Francisco Lomuto (1945)
Sin dejar rastros	Francisco Lomuto (1927, 1939)

If, in your extended tango reading, you encounter the name Pancho Laguna then be aware that it was a pseudonym for Francisco Lomuto that he occasionally used for his performances and his compositions.

José Martínez

José Martínez, born in 1890, appears in the stories of pioneers Francisco Canaro, Roberto Firpo, Augusto Berto, and Eduardo Arolas but he also deserves a separate mention because he was not simply a pianist supporting the music of others. During the years 1911 to 1918 he was a formative pioneer of the developing sound of tango dance music. He led his own trio with Osvaldo Fresedo (bandoneón) and Rafael Rinaldi (violin) then secured a contract to play at the famous Montmartre cabaret in the city centre, recruiting as second violinist Francisco Canaro. Canaro later described this as his orchestra but the billing clearly put José first: 'Martínez-Canaro'. Martínez already had a large following of tango fans and so in 1917 he was the obvious choice to be one of the two pianists[85] in the 1917 supersize carnival orchestra in Rosario. He continued with Canaro until the end of the decade when Canaro (by then the more dominant leader of the orchestra) replaced him with the tango novice Luis Riccardi, much to the loud dissatisfaction of the many Martínez followers. Nevertheless Martínez remained in vogue as an influential tango musician, as confirmed in December 1922 when he appeared on the front cover of the monthly magazine *Canciones Populares* (Popular Songs).

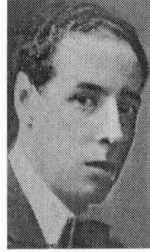

He composed many tangos some of which are still well-known today:

---

[85] the other was Roberto Firpo

COMPOSITION	BEST KNOWN RECORDED VERSION
Canaro	Francisco Canaro (1927, 1935, 1952), Juan D'Arienzo (1941), Rodolfo Biagi (1962)
La torcacita	Enrique Rodríguez (1940), Carlos Di Sarli (1941)
No aflojes, corazon	Osvaldo Fresedo (1936)

He retired from performing in 1928, aged 39, just missing out on the dawning of electric recording technology that provided most of the preserved music for today's tango dancers.

José María Rizutti

José María Rizzuti was born in 1897 in the barrio of San Cristóbal and was brought up in the world of popular music. His father was the leader of the Buenos Aires Police Band and had been making Victor gramophone recordings since 1902, including in 1908 the tangos *El choclo*, *El porteñito*, and *Gran Hotel Victoria*.

In 1917 Rizutti made his debut as the pianist in the tango quintet of bandoneonist Juan Guido with violinist Agesilao Ferrazzano. He moved from there to play in the quartet of Ricardo Brignolo which is where he first met (and started a long lasting friendship with) violinist Julio De Caro. In 1918, thanks to De Caro's recommendation, he joined the group of the star bandoneonist Eduardo Arolas.

In 1919 Rizutti and De Caro (having left Arolas) met up with Pedro Maffia (who in turn had just left Roberto Firpo) and they formed their own quartet with a second violinist. In order to convince the owner of the Café del Parque that they were a respectable group of musicians they nominated Rizzuti to do the negotiations. Rizutti dressed and spoke well and had the air of a gentleman to assure the owner, who was harbouring a stereotypical mistrust of tango musicians. Despite filling the café with customers, their relationship with the owner was tense as he rewarded them only with free coffees and water. One night a customer entered specifically to listen to Rizzuti - it was the bandoneonist Osvaldo Fresedo who was pleased with what he heard and offered him a position. Rizzuti honourably told Fresedo that he would accept only if both De Caro and Maffia could come with him. Fresedo agreed.

On 1 July 1919 Rizutti was in Osvaldo Fresedo's first sextet at the Casino Pigalle in Buenos Aires together with Pedro Maffia (briefly before he returned to Firpo), lead violinist Juan Koller supported by Julio De Caro, and double bassist Hugo Baralis[86]. Rizutti stayed with Fresedo, on and off, for another 8 years.

Rizzuti was also a respected composer of tangos including:

COMPOSITION	BEST KNOWN RECORDED VERSIONS
Adios para siempre	Osvaldo Fresedo (1936), Ángel D'Agostino (1942), Enrique Rodríguez (1943)
El cisne	Juan D'Arienzo (1938)
Milonga	Francisco Canaro (1933)
Besame en la boca	Osvaldo Fresedo (1927), Alfredo de Angelis (1950)

---

[86] Baralis had earlier played with Arolas in 1913 and his son later became the regular violinist with tango orchestra leader Aníbal Troilo

In 1933 he broadened his career to include acting, in the 1933 film *Los Tres Berretines*. He can be seen at several points in the film in the familiar role of a tango pianist and composer.

Others

Prudencio Aragón

Prudencio Aragón was born in 1887 in the Belgrano barrio of Buenos Aires. From childhood his nickname was 'Yonni' (the pronunciation of the Anglo-Saxon name 'Johnny') referring to his (apparently British-like) red hair. His older brother, Pedro, taught him how to play violin and piano and introduced him to the world of tango in which he became a regular and much loved figure. The brothers performed as the Rondalla Aragón and in 1912/13 made 10 recordings on the Atlanta label.

Prudencio was a constant and popular tango performer throughout the decade and several of his compositions were recorded by the main stars of the day: Vicente Greco, Eduardo Arolas, and Antonio Guzman. In about 1919 he moved to, and remained in, Montevideo – a decision that put him outside the accelerating tango recording industry in Buenos Aires and consequently outside of today's collective tango memory. His work is occasionally heard thanks to later recordings of his compositions:

COMPOSITION	BEST KNOWN RECORDED VERSIONS
El talar	Roberto Firpo (1949), Francisco Canaro (1956)
El Pardo Cejas	Francisco Canaro (1938 and 1956)
Mate amargo	Francisco Canaro (1938)

Manuel Aróztegui

Manuel Gregorio Aróztegui was born in Montevideo, Uruguay in 1888 and within a year his parents, Manuel and Amalia, took him to live in Buenos Aires. As a boy Aróztegui was inspired to play music having heard bandoneonist Juan 'Pacho' Maglio in a café back in 1905. He first learnt how to play the mandolin and violin before developing his piano skills and was taught how to read musical notation by Carlos Hernani Macchi, the influential tango flautist and composer.

Aróztegui soon became a regular performer and began mixing with those in the tango scene. He became friends with the musician D'Agostino who invited him to his home to play tangos on the piano, the same piano upon which D'Agostino's son Ángel[87] was still learning.

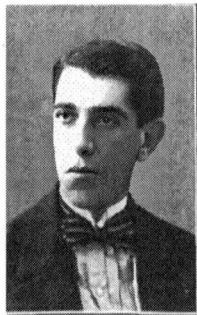

El compositor nacional don Manuel Aróztegui, que acaba de publicar «Champagne Tango», para piano.

---

[87] Ángel D'Agostino became a tango orchestra leader and recording artist in the 1940s

In 1912 he had a contract at the café El Maratón with an accompanying violinist and bandoneónist but after six months the owner decided to cease providing live tango music at his café. He was not personally averse to the music, or to the musicians, but this trio had attracted a certain crowd and after a series of rowdy disturbances a gun was pulled resulting in serious injuries. Unsettled by the firearm incident, Aróztegui found himself a more serene venue at the café of a cinema Los Cristianos. It was whilst there that he composed the tangos:

COMPOSITION	BEST KNOWN RECORDED VERSIONS
El apache argentino	Ánibal Troilo (1942), Juan D'Arienzo (1944), Roberto Firpo (1953), Francsico Canaro (1955), Alfredo De Angelis (1969)
El cachafez	Juan D'Arienzo (1937), Carlos Di Sarli (1954);
Champagne tango	Juan D'Arienzo (1938), Francisco Canaro (1938), Carlos Di Sarli (1944 and 1952).

On 6 November 1915 Aróztegui's photograph (above) was published in the magazine Caras y Caretas. The text reads 'the national composer Manuel Aróztegui who has just published Champagne tango for piano'. Although he passed away in November 1938 he lived just long enough to have heard and enjoyed the 1937 and 1938 D'Arienzo and Canaro recordings of Champagne tango.

D'Agostino

Many in the extended D'Agostino family, in the barrio of Parque Patricios, were musicians and well-connected to the tango stars of the day, particularly those who visited to gather around their home piano. In 1900 the D'Agostinos celebrated the birth of Ángel Domingo Emilio who within 6 years had already demonstrated his talents at the keyboard. Although he had heard his father and visiting friends (such as Manuel Aróztegui and Alfredo Bevilacqua) getting excited by their tangos little Ángel was not at all attracted to it and much preferred to practice the classics.

In 1911 Ángel D'Agostino was playing classical pieces and popular tunes at the piano in the children's Sunday theatre in the Palermo Zoological Gardens. By his side was his violinist friend Juan D'Arienzo, also 11 years old. The following year he was playing at parties in the grand homes of Buenos Aires and in theatre orchestras. He had widened his childhood taste from classical music towards jazz and was slowly developing his interest in tango. By 1915 he was playing at silent cinemas in a quartet, again with violinist friend Juan D'Arienzo, plus the bandoneón player Juan Deambroggio ('Bachicha') and the cellist Ennio Bolognini[88]. In 1918 after the announcement of the World War's cessation Bolognini rolled his piano out on to the balcony of his house so that Ángel D'Agostino could accompany him to the anthem of freedom over tyranny *La Marseillaise*.

Ángel D'Agostino did not gravitate towards tango until the start of the 1930s when he was in his early 30s. He would secure a contract with RCA Victor in November 1940 and his recording output for the following decade or so ensured that he still remains a favourite at today's milongas around the world.

---

[88] later acknowledged as the world's finest classical cellist, who for fun sometimes played it flamenco style like a guitar

4. Bandoneonists

Arolas, Bernstein, Berto, Brignolo, De Leone
Espósito

Eduardo Arolas

Eduardo Arolas was already an established bandoneonist and composer with a growing following of tango fans but he had realised that in order to improve he needed to study music theory. In 1911, at the age of 19, he began his studies at the conservatory of José Bombig, leader of the Buenos Aires Prison Service Band. There he learnt music theory and notation whilst at the same time continuing to perform alongside changing line-ups that included the cool, string-slapping guitarist Leopoldo Thompson, the spark-inducing violinist 'El Pibe' Ernesto Ponzio, the serious pianists Agustín Bardi and Prudencio Aragón, and his future drinking companion violinist David 'Tito' Roccatagliata. In 1913 Arolas was performing in the provinces where he met and fell in love with Delia López who accompanied him back to Buenos Aires. That year he was invited in to the new Odeon recording facilities of Max Glücksmann at the Casa Lepage. Recording as the Orquesta Típica Criolla Arolas (a quartet with a guitar, violin, and flute) he completed over 30 tracks included his own compositions :

- *Una noche de garufa* (named after the café at which he regularly played)*;*
- *Delia* (his tribute to his lover), and

131

- *El Rey de los bordoneos* (his tribute to Gracione De Leone's days as a guitarist).

He also recorded Rosendo Mendizábal's *El entrerriano* and *Viento en popa*, Alfredo Bevilacqua's *Gran muñeca*, Vicente Greco's *Estoy penando*, Prudencio Aragon's *Las siete palabras* and three bandoneón solos. In some of the tangos you can hear the earliest appearance of what became the traditional tango two-note ending that has become known as the 'chan chan'. Arolas did not invent tango's signature ending (there is a hint of it in Vicente Greco's 1912 recording *Vicentito*) but his recordings are certainly the first to regularly finish in that way.

Buenos Aires, 19 de marzo 1914.

Sr. D. Max Glücksmann.

Muy señor mío:

Dirijo a Vd. la presente para manifestarle que los discos «Odeón», impresionados por mi, tanto solos de Bandonión como acompañados por orquesta típica criolla, son los que me han dejado más satisfecho.

La reproducción es perfecta, y en ella se reconoce la ejecución original con toda fidelidad.

Como lleve la matriz original, mi firma resulta grabada en cada disco; y eso le da garantía de que es auténtico.

Saludo a Vd. con toda consideración.

Eduardo Arolas

In 1914 he recorded on other labels[89] (Arena, Polydor, Premier, Sonora and Oro-phon) and like many other bands his was often described as an 'orquesta criolla' although it varied in formation between a quartet, quintet, and sextet. On Orophon he recorded as the Orquesta Típica Porteña although the digital transfers today make no mention of Porteña only to Eduardo Arolas. On 19

---

[89] the labelling of recordings did not necessarily indicate different, competing commercial enterprises

March 1914 he wrote to Max Glücksmann declaring that the
Odeon discs of his solos on bandoneón, as well as those of his
orquesta típica, were the recordings that had left him most satisfied.
The reproduction perfectly reflected the original performance with
total fidelity and as he had signed the master recording his
signature appeared on every recording, guaranteeing its
authenticity.

Amongst his 20 or more recordings in 1914 were tangos that are
still well-known today mainly due to the versions by later
orchestras:

TITLE	BEST KNOWN RECORDED VERSIONS
La viruta	Juan D'Arienzo (1937), Francisco Canaro (1938), Carlos Di Sarli (1943, 1952), Rodolfo Biagi (1948)
El choclo	Orquesta Típica Victor (1929), Juan D'Arienzo and Francisco Canaro (both 1937), Osvaldo Fresedo (1939), Roberto Firpo (1940), Ángel D'Agostino (1941)
Germaine	Carlos Di Sarli (1941, 1951, 1955), Roberto Firpo (1940)
Marejada	Roberto Firpo (1932), Orquesta Típica Victor (1937), Carlos Di Sarli (1941)

These were his golden years - he was in high demand as a
bandoneonist, composer, and as a tango personality. In 1916 he
was performing both with his own quintet and guesting in the
orchestras of others, on both sides of the Río de la Plata. At the
start of 1917 in carnival season he was in the formidable line up of
the giant Firpo-Canaro orchestra in Rosario. The poster for the
event included photographs of the main musicians and, as one

might expect, featured those of Firpo and Canaro more prominently than the others. But in the centre and between the two leaders was the photograph of Eduardo Arolas. The position suggests an elevated status of Arolas and although we do not know the names of the 200 tangos that they played it is more than likely that they included several compositions of Arolas which by that time included *Una noche de garufa, Derecho viejo, Rawson, La guitarrita,* and (jointly composed with Firpo) *Fuegos artificiales.* Later as part of the same continuing carnival season Arolas was performing at dances in the best hotels in a trio with David Tito Roccatagliata and the pianist Juan Carlos Cobían.

In April 1917 visiting engineers from the Victor Talking Machine Company (George Cheney and Charles Althouse) had set up their portable recording equipment in the premises of the leading Victor distribution agent Pratt, 205-217 Calle San Martin. Over the course of six days in April and May Arolas and his musicians visited and made 29 recordings. Although labelled as an orquesta típica the quintet comprised of Arolas on the bandoneón, Carlos Lombardo and Rafael Tuegols on violin, Luis Riccardi[90] on piano, and an unnamed cellist. On some of the recordings Arolas used the cello as an alternative to the double bass. On 23 April 1917, whilst setting up to record the North American rhythm of *In the Land of Harmony*, the tight timetable of the Victor engineers was thrown in to disarray. Cheney and Althouse annotated the ledger 'cellist forgot music and delayed duty by one hour'. Also on some recordings the piano was replaced by a guitar and although the guitarist is not named it is likely to have been Riccardi switching instruments. The engineers' side comments in the company ledger offer some further revealing moments. On 23 April they were

---

[90] the future long term pianist of Francisco Canaro from the 1920s to 1960s

clearly impressed by the recording of the Arolas composition *Rawson* and noted it as 'an important number'. They were not wrong as it is a tango still enjoyed today thanks to the later recordings by Juan D'Arienzo. They were less impressed on 26 April when, having recorded 5 tracks, they brought the day to an early close by writing 'stopped for want of good stuff'. It is unlikely that Arolas had run out of good material but perhaps the musicians were tired and not able to satisfy the engineers' expectations. On 15 May the singer Francisco Bianco arrived to record with the Arolas quintet that resulted in further unhappiness[91]. The next day was a new start and so prior to committing to the recording of the vals *Blanca nieve* Cheney and Althouse decided to have a test performance particularly as Arolas had brought along a harp. His innovation was abandoned with the single word in the ledger 'disappointment'. The harp however did make a return to the world of tango in the 1930s line-up of Osvaldo Fresedo's orquesta típica and became Fresedo's signature sound for many years thereafter.

On Saturday 6 October 1917 the community hall Centro Gallego in the barrio of Avellaneda (where it still stands today) was holding its Grand Artistic Festival and Family Dance event. The advertisement declared it to be 'In honour of the famous bandoneonist and national composer Eduardo Arolas'. The neighbouring barrios of Avellenada, Barracas, and La Boca all considered Arolas to be a local boy and so his presence, playing his tangos for the people of Avellenada, would have been a mutual honour.

---

[91] see *Singers/Bianco* above

The tango compositions of Arolas were innovative and energetic and many are still regularly heard at today's milongas:

COMPOSITION	BEST KNOWN RECORDED VERSIONS
Comme il faut	Juan D'Arienzo (1936); Aníbal Troilo as his first ever recording (1938), Carlos Di Sarli (1947, 1951, and 1955)
Una noche de garufa	Carlos Di Sarli (1931), Ricardo Tanturi (1941), Francisco Canaro (1953)
Derecho viejo	Francisco Canaro (1927, 1938), Juan D'Arienzo (1939, 1948), Osvaldo Fresedo (1941), Osvaldo Pugliese (1945)
La cachila	Carlos Di Sarli (1941, 1952), Osvaldo Fresedo (1932), Osvaldo Pugliese (1945)
Retintín	Francisco Canaro (1927, 1938), Juan D'Arienzo (1936)
Rawson	Juan D'Arienzo (1936, 1947)
La guitarrita	Carlos Di Sarli (1928), Francisco Canaro (1930), Juan D'Arienzo (1936), Miguel Caló (1949)
Papas calientes	Edgardo Donato (1937), Juan D'Arienzo (1967)
Lagrimas	Ricardo Tanturi (1941), Juan D'Arienzo (1947)
Mishiadura	Edgardo Donato (1942)
Catamarca	Carlos Di Sarli (1940), Francisco Lomuto (1943), Julio De Caro (1940)
El Marne	Orquesta Típica Victor (1933), Juan D'Arienzo (1939, 1950, 1954), Aníbal Troilo (1952), Osvaldo Pugliese (1969)
La Cachila	Osvaldo Fresedo (1927, 1932), Carlos Di Sarli (1941, 1952), Osvaldo Pugliese (1945, 1952)

In 1915 Arolas composed *Comme Il Faut* with guitarist Rafael Iriarte who in 1917 submitted the same tango under the name *Comparsa Criolla*. Listen to the versions of *Comme Il Faut* by Juan D'Arienzo

(1936) and by Aníbal Troilo (1938) and then listen to *Comparsa Criolla* by Ricardo Tanturi (1941). They are more or less the same tango with two names and two separately registered composers.

Eduardo Arolas changed the course of danceable tango music. His sound was an inspiration and influencer of the music of Julio De Caro and Osvaldo Fresedo and therefore those that flowed from them (such as Pedro Laurenz, Aníbal Troilo, and Osvaldo Pugliese). Arolas slowed tango music down. Other bandoneonists (like Juan Maglio, Augusto Berto, Arturo Bernstein, Genaro Espósito, and Vicente Greco) did the same. The reason for the slower pace is likely to have been a mix of artistic choice and a result of the bandoneonists' limited dexterity on this difficult instrument. Both Julio De Caro and Pedro Maffia have each credited Arolas with creating a new tango sound on the bandoneón by being the first (I would rather say 'by being amongst the first') to slur the notes and by making the instrument 'groan'. They also credited him with the 'arrastre' (a percussive slide effect) that Roberto Firpo is said to have imitated on his piano. They are honouring Arolas and so we should not take the compliments as fact, for example it is highly likely that guitarists earler than Arolas had also deployed the arrastre.

The Arolas connection with Julio de Caro is interesting because not only did he contribute to luring the young Julio away from his family home (contrary to the wishes of De Caro's father) but he also heavily influenced Julio's understanding of the structure of tango music. Julio De Caro is regularly credited with changing the direction of tango towards more elaborate arrangements but it would be fairer to say that he continued the innovations of Eduardo Arolas, Juan Carlos Cobián, and Osvaldo Fresedo who changed the fast 2/4 rhythm of the tango to a slower, deeper, and wider 4/8 construction. During those years Arolas further developed his sound by introducing instruments that were not traditionally linked to tango - a 1916 photograph shows the Arolas musicians with drums and a cello. In his live performances (but not recordings) he included the harp, a saxophone and a banjo to spark the public's interest and create a point of difference between him and other orquestas típicas. His sound experiments bring to mind the later Francisco Canaro who added interest with the musical saw, the trumpet, and the organ.

The demand for Arolas was growing to such an extent that his quartet was performing twice a day at different venues. At that time it was usual practice for musicians to frequently join and leave orchestras, rather than to stay on fixed period contracts, and so a number of musicians (who later became leading tango stars in their own right) had the benefit of playing under the guidance of Eduardo Arolas. Arolas recruited the 18-year-old violinist Julio De Caro. Within weeks he also needed a replacement pianist and De Caro recommended his friend José María Rizzuti. Shortly afterwards a new bandoneonist arrived, Manuel Pizarro, who later became one of the tango pioneers in Paris. Experience with Arolas benefitted many future tango stars.

In the next few years Eduardo Arolas experienced extreme bouts of both creativity and personal destruction. He discovered that the two most precious people in his life, his brother Enrique and his lover Delia, had not only been having an affair whilst he was away on tour but that she was also pregnant with Enrique's baby. Distraught, Arolas escaped to Montevideo. Whilst there he played at the annual carnival in an octet of three bandoneóns (Arolas, Genaro Espósito, and José Quevado), three violins (Rafael Tuegols, Julio De Caro, and Julio González), a piano (José María Rizzuti) and a violincello. He also joined the quintet of the local bandleader Carlos Warren at the prestigious Parque Hotel and in the line up was violinist Edgardo Donato who recalled that the dancers on that occasion stopped to turn towards Arolas in complete admiration of his mastery of the bandoneón. He became so influential and popular that by August 1919 the quintet had become known as the Arolas-Warren orchestra. He was still the 'Tiger of the Bandoneón' despite the chaos and sadness of his private life. Forever seeking female company Arolas found some solace for his heartbreak in the arms of the French Alice Lesage and when he received an offer to perform in Paris he took it.

Following the ever-increasing tango success of Arolas from 1909 to 1919, the next four years would be the worst, and last, years of his life[92].

I recommend that you watch the 1951 film *Derecho Viejo* based on the life of Eduardo Arolas. The scenes are credible enough and include 'Arolas' playing his compositions *Una noche de garufa*, *Derecho viejo*, *La Cachila*, and *Retintín*.

---

[92] see *Get To Know the Tango Pioneers 1920 to 1935*

Arturo Bernstein

Arturo Bernstein had been a favourite solo bandoneonist in the Buenos Aires barrio of La Boca since the start of the century. Between 1913 and 1915 he recorded over 40 tracks as El Aleman[93] Quinteto Criollo on the Atlanta label. Like other advertised Atlanta quintets his was in reality a quartet of bandoneón, guitar, violin, and flute. Why name a quartet as a quintet? There were two compatible reasons:

- the group was a quintet but the missing musician on the recordings was the pianist. Recording engineers had difficulty (with their portable equipment and limitations of their make-shift recording rooms) to balance the powerful sound of the piano with the other instruments;
- a quintet had more marketing *gravitas* than a quartet.

To ensure that Bernstien reached a wider buying public he included many other popular rhythms such as polka, mazurkas, chacarera, gato, and zamacuecas. Tango to Arturo, and to many of his admiring fans, was just another one of the beautiful national *aires* and not considered to be a specialist nor unique genre. You can listen to a selection of Arturo's recordings on most music streaming services and I particularly recommend the popular tangos *El caburé*, *El pollito*, *Tinta verde*, *Cordón de oro*, *Canaro*, and *Didi*.

Arturo was a pioneer who has fallen from today's collective memory because his recordings are no longer heard and he did not leave any compositions that were recorded by the later orchestras. However he remained a giant in the tango world that culminated in 1935 with a performance on Radio del Pueblo in a nostalgic

---

[93] his parents were German immigrants (from Brazil)

sextet (that also included Enrique Saborido on piano, Vicente Pecci on flute, Vicente Pepe on violin, and two guitarists). He died in September that year and, as a measure of the high regard in which he was held, his fans organised a benefit concert to raise funds to support his family. Amongst the many tango stars who played in that concert were the big name orchestra leaders Francisco Canaro, Edgardo Donato, and Osvaldo Fresedo; the singers Ernesto Famá, Andrés Falgás, Teófilo Ibáñez; and bandoneonist Ciriaco Ortiz. They recognised Bernstein's contribution to tango music and accordingly paid tribute to him.

Augusto Berto

Augusto Berto was born in Bahía Blanca in 1889 and moved to Buenos Aires with his family five years later. He taught himself guitar and mandolin, both being common instruments among Italian immigrant families, and by the age of 14 in 1903 he had progressed to playing violin in the local orchestra. However there was another instrument that excited Augusto more than the violin. Growing up in the barrio of Villa Crespo he had plenty of opportunity to see the new bandoneonists such as Sebastián Ramos Mejía, Domingo Santa Cruz, and Pablo Romero. One of his local cafés, La Morocha, had its own bandoneón for players to come and use and one such local player was José 'Pepino' Piazza. Fascinated by the sound and energy of those visiting musicians Berto took lessons from Pepino, who a few years later also taught Pedro Maffia[94]. In 1906 Berto started to perform alongside Pepino at La Morocha and other local cafés until branching out beyond

---

[94] Pedro Maffia in the 1920s influenced the direction of tango music towards a greater sophistication and complexity.

his teacher's guiding hands. He composed a tango firmly based on a traditional country tune that he regularly played but did not name for many years. *La payanca* was first recorded by the orquesta típica of Eduardo Arolas in 1917 supporting the payador singer Francisco Blanco, thereby blending together folk and tango stars. *La payanca* is best known to us today thanks to the recordings by the Orquesta Típica Victor (1926), Juan D'Arienzo (1936, 1949, 1954), Roberto Firpo (1946), Francisco Canaro (1964), and Osvaldo Pugliese (1964).

Berto formed a trio with violinist Francisco Canaro[95] and guitarist Domingo Salerno in 1912. He did not know that at one of their performances in a café-bar in Palermo a 15-year-old customer was watching him intently. Augusto Berto inspired that boy to become one of the outstanding bandoneonists, orchestra leaders, and tango recording stars over the following 50 years. That boy was Osvaldo Fresedo and we will find out more about him later in this section. Also in 1912 Berto was contracted to play at the Café del los Loros and increased his trio to a quintet by recruiting flautist José Fuster and second bandoneonist Vicente Loduca. In late 1912 he and his new quintet posed for a photographer (below) with Berto seated in the centre. He still had his original guitarist Domingo Salerno (seated right) but everyone else had changed. Canaro had left to join the sextet of Vicente Greco and so was replaced by Julio Doutry (seated left). Berto had dispensed with a second bandoneón, recruited a replacement flautist Luis Teisseire and added the pianist José Martínez (standing without an instrument as the photographer's studio did not have a piano). They recorded 10

---

[95] who he had first met as a fellow painter and decorator at the newly completed Congress building

tracks as the Quinteto Criollo on the Atlanta label but only four musicians were on the recordings: sometimes Martínez on piano and sometimes Salerno on guitar. The piano and guitar together did not work well in the recording process and so either one or the other was dropped. Two compositions of Martínez are the only tangos from that session that are familiar to us today (due to the recordings made by later orchestras):

COMPOSITION	BEST KNOWN RECORDED VERSIONS
El pensamiento	Adolfo Carabelli (1932), Julio De Caro (1942), Juan D'Arienzo (1945), Roberto Firpo (1956)
La torcacita	Enrique Rodríguez (1940), Carlos Di Sarli (1941), Juan D'Arienzo (1971)

In 1913/14 Berto returned to Atlanta and recorded as the

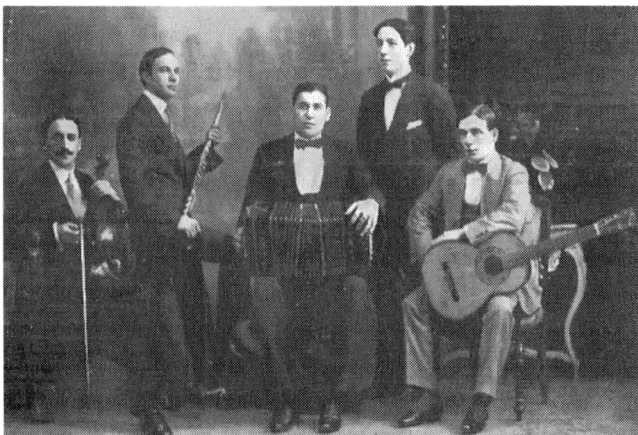

Quinteto Criollo Augusto. He recorded a further 100 tracks. I do recommend that you listen to the Atlanta recordings that are available on CD and most music streaming services. They are reasonably well preserved, upbeat, and entertaining.

Augusto Berto's reputation, and his following, grew continuously and in 1917 he signed other recording contracts with both Columbia and Victor. On 3 May 1917 Berto's quintet entered the large department store of Pratt on the Calle San Martin and headed for the room especially adapted by the two visiting Victor recording engineers George Cheney and Charles Althouse. Over two days they recorded 20 tracks including Berto's most famous tango composition *La payanca* but the second day did not run as smoothly as the first. It took a while for them to start the day and the engineers noted the reason as 'Lost one hour waiting for the fluter'. Then a violin string snapped but a gut replacement could not be found and so a lesser quality wire string was fitted. Finally for some reason the engineers were not happy with the clash in tones between the flute and the piano on their zamba track and so switched the piano for a guitar 'Piano out, guitar in. Decided flute doing harm'. Sadly nearly all of the tangos recorded are now no longer familiar to us yet it is reasonable to assume that Berto chose to record those particular ones because they had proven to be popular at his performances. Fortunately there are some Berto compositions that we can enjoy today through the recordings of others:

COMPOSITION	BEST KNOWN RECORDED VERSIONS
La payanca	Orquesta Típica Victor (1926), Juan D'Arienzo (1936, 1949, 1954), Roberto Firpo (1946), Francisco Canaro (1964), Osvaldo Pugliese (1964)
Don Esteban	Juan D'Arienzo (1936), Francisco Canaro (1927, 1938), Roberto Firpo (1942)
Belén	Carlos Di Sarli (1929), Edgardo Donato (1936)
Donde estás corazón	Francisco Canaro, Julio De Caro, Orquesta Típica Victor (all in 1930)
Penas de amor	Juan D'Arienzo (1935)

As a sign of respect by other composers he was the recipient of several dedications on their published sheet music, including *El triunfo* by Francisco Canaro and *Quejas de bandoneón* by Juan de Dios Filberto.

Berto continued to perform and in the 1930s he regularly conducted a tango orchestra with guest singers that included Ángel Vargas (yet to find fame with Ángel D'Agostino). Additionally from 1926 to the early 1930s the magazine *Caras y Caretas* carried advertisements for bandoneóns and included assurances that the bandoneón model had been checked and validated by Augusto Berto. There could have been no finer guarantee.

Ricardo Brignolo

Ricardo Luis Brignolo was born in 1892 in Buenos Aires and in 1911/1912 he passed by a café-bar in the barrio of La Boca and heard music coming from within. He entered and listened in fascination to the instrument being played. When the piece had finished Brignolo asked whether the musician might give him lessons. Genaro Espósito was not interested. He may have been a leading tango bandoneonist but he was not a teacher nor was he a trained musician: he did not understand music theory and barely understood how he himself had intuitively learnt to master his instrument. Despite repeated refusals Brignolo persisted and Espósito eventually agreed to teach him the rudiments.

In 1913 Brignolo was good enough, and bold enough[96], to stand in for Espósito at the Bar Iglesias on the Calle Corrientes and play alongside the pianist Roberto Firpo. From 1914 he was leading his own groups and playing in café-bars and cinemas across the city. By the end of the decade he was playing in the orchestras of others (pianists Carlos Vicente Geroni Flores, Juan Carlos Cobían, and Samuel Castriota) and in the 1920s would lead his own orchestra and record on the Brunswick label.

Graciano De Leone

A regular in the cafés of the barrio of La Boca during this period was guitarist Graciano De Leone. In 1909 he had accompanied the novice bandoneonist Eduardo Arolas and by 1910 and 1911 had himself switched to the bandoneón and was playing at the Café

---

[96] his nickname appropriately became Ricardo the Lion Heart

Royal (known locally as Café Griego) with violinist Eduardo Monelos.

In 1912 De Leone's quartet played at the Café Argentino with violinist David 'Tito' Roccatagliata, flautist Carlos Hernani Macchi, and pianist Agustín Bardi - all of whom were major contributors to, and influencers of, the tango music that is enjoyed today. Also in 1912 Eduardo Arolas composed and published the tango *El Rey de los bordoneos* and dedicated it to De Leone in recognition of his mastery of his guitar strum. The dedication is both a useful insight in to the tango style of De Leone's playing and a measure of the high regard in which he was held.

From 1913 to 1919 De Leone played in very many combinations of musicians: in the Café La Buseca, in the barrio Avellenada, with pianist Agustín Bardi and guitarist Ricardo 'Mochila' González (who later also changed his instrument for the bandoneón, encouraged by De Leone); at the prestigious cabaret Armenonville in Palermo with pianist Juan Carlos Cobían;

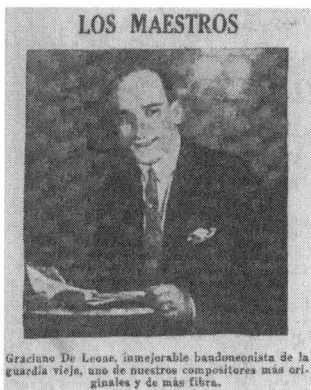

LOS MAESTROS

Graciano De Leone, inmejorable bandoneonista de la guardia vieja, uno de nuestros compositores más originales y de más fibra.

at high class hotels such as the Tigre Hotel and Club; and with pianist Francisco De Caro at the seaside resort Mar del Plata. He was also the regular performer at the famous Bar Domínguez and was later immortalised in the opening poem of the tango *Café Domínguez* (recorded by Ángel D'Agostino in 1955). The poem starts '*Café Domínguez de la vieja calle Corrientes que ya no queda, café del cuarteto bravo de Graciano de Leone a tus mesas caian Pirincho, Arola, Firpo y*

Pacho a escuchar tus tangos' (Café Domínguez in the old Corrientes street that no longer exists, the café of the magnificent quartet of Graciano De Leone where Canaro (Pirincho), Arolas, Firpo, and Maglio (Pacho) came to listen to your tangos).

De Leone continued to perform and to compose through the 1920s and 1930s. His compositions that we still hear today, thanks to the recordings of others, are:

COMPOSITION	BEST KNOWN RECORDED VERSIONS
Reliquias porteñas	recorded as a milonga by Francisco Canaro (1938)
Un tierra negra	Juan D'Arienzo, Roberto Firpo, Francisco Canaro (1942), Carlo Di Sarli (1943 and 1953)
Un lamento	Carlos Di Sarli (1929, 1944, 1953), Ángel D'Agostino and Roberto Firpo (both in 1942)

Un Lamento is an excellent tango to compare different versions across the decades. As well as the better known recordings also listen to the recordings by Ferrer-Filipotto (1917), by singer Ignacio Corsini (1920), by the Quinteto Los Virtuosos[97] (1936), by Osvaldo Pugliese (1960), and finally by Juan D'Arienzo (1969).

On 10 May 1924 the magazine *Caras y Caretas* published a three-page article entitled 'The Maestros of the Bandoneón' and the first page included a photograph of Graciano De Leone. On 14 May 1928 (above) the magazine *Canción Moderna* celebrated him as a

---

[97] bandoneonists Pedro Maffia and Ciriaco Ortiz, violinists Elvino Vardaro and Julio De Caro, and pianist Francisco De Caro

maestro 'the unbeatable bandoneonist of the *guardia vieja*, one of our most original composers'.

He is today one of those pioneers whose name is largely unknown and yet he was clearly highly respected during his lifetime and for some decades afterwards. I hope that his inclusion in this book can go some way towards re-establishing his memory amongst today's tango fans.

Genaro Espósito

The 1895 census shows that Francisco and Ana Espósito were Italian immigrants settled in San Telmo with five children: Salvador, Genaro (born in 1886), Carmen, Arturo, and Carlos. Francisco and Ana co-owned a general store[98] in partnership with Antonio Solari who was a butcher and a bandoneón player. Solari entertained the customers with his instrument that was ostentatiously adorned with golden edges. In his early adolescence Genaro Espósito was working at the general store, listening to Solari and his accompanying musicians, and learning guitar, piano, and the basics of the bandoneón. He first started performing at his parent's store and then ventured to other bars and cafés where he developed a loyal following. He was known locally for being able to replicate the sounds of the universally familiar and well-loved street organitos, in a sense changing the relationship with the organito that had previously replaced live musicians. At one of his usual café-bars in the Suarez and Necochea corner of La Boca a young

---

[98] that also provided tables and entertainment, similar to a café

man (Ricardo Brignolo) heard him playing and, fascinated by the sound, waited until the performance was over to ask him for lessons. Today Brignolo is himself considered to have been an early tango pioneer and so this line of Brignolo learning from Espósito learning from Solari who may have learnt from others unknown is a clear example of the longer, often unappreciated, tango story.

Returning to Genaro Espósito, now newly married[99] he needed to maintain a reliable income so was in full-time employment during the day at a machinery importer based in San Telmo. In 1910 his wife gave birth to a son, Francisco Teodoro[100], yet despite his domestic responsibilities Genaro Espósito did not abandon his love for tango music and played when he could, successfully catching the attention of more than one recording company.

From January to March 1912 two engineers, Henry Hagen and Charles Althouse, from the North American Victor Talking Machine Company were in Buenos Aires with portable recording equipment to capture local artists. Amongst them was the quartet of Genaro Espósito (bandoneón) with Julio Doutry (violin), Félix Camarano (guitar), and José Fuster (usually a flautist but on these sessions he played a clarinet). They recorded 15 tracks that were released as 10 doubled-sided discs augmented by 5 'B' sides that did not feature them at all but were of other various artists such as the singer guitarist Ignacio Corsini[101], the folk and classical guitarist Juan Ríos, a solo accordionist, and a mazurka band. On one of

---

[99] the best man at his wedding was friend, neighbour, and so-called 'Father of Tango' Ángel Villoldo

[100] who followed his father in to the tango music business by becoming the stand-in pianist for the Canaro orchestra and later in the 1940s led his own Orquesta Típica Tano Genaro.

[101] including Corsini's first ever recording, Juan Maglio's vals composition *Violetas* (better known now by Alberto Castillo's 1948 version).

those records it was Espósito's tango on the B-side whilst Corsini was presented on the A. It appears that Victor at that time was not fully confident that the record buying public was entirely ready for a whole disc of Genaro Espósito.

The tangos that Espósito chose to record were clearly those that were already popular in 1912 but only a few of which are still familiar today:

TITLE	BEST KNOWN RECORDED VERSIONS
Felicia	by Osvaldo Fresedo (1927), Francisco Canaro (1929), Roberto Firpo (1937), Juan D'Arienzo (1939)
El irresistible	Francisco Lomuto (1931), Juan D'Arienzo (1936), Francisco Canaro (1939), Osvaldo Fresedo (1943), Rodolfo Biagi (1946)
Francia (a vals)	Juan D'Arienzo (1935), Francisco Canaro (1943).

With regard to the other tangos it is a great pity, as ever with the repertoire of the pioneers, that so many fine tangos were not given a new boost of life by the later orchestras using more modern recording methods.

In 1912 Espósito recorded again but that time with Columbia and with him were pianist Roberto Firpo and violinist David 'Tito' Roccatagliata. From examining the labels it appears that Columbia was unsure how to categorise them because each label carried two separate descriptive terms simultaneously: 'orquesta típica' and 'orquesta criolla'. Furthermore Columbia got in to a muddle with Espósito's name, misspelling it as Orquesta Típica Gennaro and on one label mysteriously putting it in inverted commas as Orquesta

Típica "Genaro". You can listen to 6 of those recordings on the website of DAHR[102].

In the same year (1912) Espósito was at the Café La Marina at the corner of Suarez and Necochea in La Boca with Alcides Palavecino on violin and the North American pianist Harold Phillips. Phillips was principally a jazz and, more recently, a cake-walk specialist and so today we can only imagine the exciting swing that he gave to their tangos. Who knows what his influence may have been on the Buenos Aires tango scene had he not decided to travel to Europe the following year, devastatingly timing his arrival in Belgium at the same time as the advancing German army. Phillips is believed to have been arrested, accused of being an American spy and executed by firing squad. Meanwhile back in the Café La Marina Espósito was facing his own volley of bullets. Next door to the café there was a political meeting, probably a group of anarchists. La Boca at that time was a hot bed of unrest and rebellion. The meeting degenerated in to a brawl and spilled in to the street where pistols were drawn. Inside La Marina the band played on until a stray bullet came flying through the glass window and punctured the bandoneón on Espósito's lap[103].

In 1912/13 Espósito was the leader of the resident quartet at Bar Iglesias on the Calle Corrientes, the favourite meeting place for the emerging tango musicians. The pianist was Roberto Firpo and the violinists were Ernesto Zambonini and Alcides Palavecino. His quartet recorded on the labels of ERA and Artigas. Amongst the couple of dozen recordings were Espósito's two bandoneón solos,

---

[102] Discography of American Historical Recordings
[103] as recalled by Genaro Espósito himself but of course possibly elaborated for the value of a good tale

perhaps inspired by Maglio's successful solo bandoneón recording the year before. Many of the recorded tangos are still well-known to us today thanks to versions by later orchestras such as:

TITLE	BEST KNOWN RECORDED VERSIONS
Pinta Brava	Francisco Canaro (1933)
El Gavilan	Francisco Canaro (1930)
El apache argentino	Juan D'Arienzo (1944), Aníbal Troilo (1944), Francisco Canaro (1955)
El cachafaz	Juan D'Arienzo (1937), Carlos Di Sarli (1954)
Una fija	Miguel Caló (1951), Carlos Di Sarli (1954 & 1958)
Union Cívica	Juan D'Arienzo (1938), Rodolfo Biagi (1938)
Sentimiento criollo	Carlos Di Sarli (1941)

Espósito switched to the Atlanta label as the 'Quinteto Criollo Tano Genaro' and released over 20 tangos including four bandoneón solos and a sprinkling of vals, mazurkas, and polka. The chosen tangos most known to us today are:

TITLE	BEST KNOWN RECORDED VERSIONS
El entrerriano	Francisco Canaro (1927, 1929, 1952), Osvaldo Fresedo (1927, 1944), Orquesta Típica Victor (1927), Roberto Firpo (1937), Rodolfo Biagi (1941), Juan D'Arienzo (1946), Aníbal Troilo (1944)
Viento en popa	Francisco Canaro (1937), Roberto Firpo (1948)
Rodríguez Peña	Francisco Canaro (1927 & 1938), Osvaldo Fresedo (1927 & 1942),

	Orquesta Típica Victor (1927), Roberto Firpo (1937), Juan D'Arienzo (1938), Carlos Di Sarli (1952 & 1956)
Lagrimas y sonrias	Juan D'Arienzo (1936), Rodolfo Biagi (1941)

In late 1913 the restaurant cabaret Armenonville organised a competition to find a resident tango band. Amongst the many contestants were Juan Maglio's quartet and the Espósito Trio. Surprisingly the Armenonville chose none of them but made an offer only to the pianist of the Espósito Trio - Roberto Firpo - and asked him to form his own quartet. Espósito was therefore left without a pianist and as a result the Espósito 'Quintet' returned to record a dozen tracks on the Atlanta label as a quartet of bandoneón, guitar rather than piano, violin and flute. Shortly afterwards Eduardo Arolas suggested to Espósito that he should try a new pianist from Bahía Blanca who was playing at a silent cinema. Espósito found him, liked him, and took him on - the pianist's name was Juan Carlos Cobían, soon to be one of the great tango composers and personalities. Cobían was not like the typical tango musician with whom Espósito normally worked - he was refined in his manners, his speech, his clothing, and his music. The young 18-year-old Cobían was not comfortable playing with the musically illiterate Genaro Espósito and the often drunk and obnoxious Zambonini in the rough bars and cafés of Buenos Aires. He soon departed thereby leaving Espósito once more without a pianist. After finding a pianist for a tour in Cordoba in 1915 Espósito then recruited the 17-year-old Vicente Gorrese who stayed with Espósito for two years and much later went on to play on the recordings of the Orquesta Típica Victor from 1925 to 1931 as well as on Juan D'Arienzo's first recordings in 1928.

In 1918 Espósito made four double-sided recordings on the Telephone label (the short-lived successor to Atlanta) that included *Catamarca*, composed by Eduardo Arolas, that is still familiar today thanks to the later recordings by Francisco Lomuto (1931), Carlos Di Sarli (1939), and Julio De Caro (1940).

Genaro Espósito had been performing since 1900, recording since 1912, and in 1919 was amongst the big names and rising stars on both sides of the Río de la Plata, appearing at the Montevideo carnival alongside bandoneonists Eduardo Arolas and Carlos Warren, violinist Julio De Caro, and pianist José María Rizutti. In the 1920s and 1930s he would be at the height of his performing and recording success - neither in Buenos Aires nor Montevideo but in Europe (mainly Paris).

Osvaldo Fresedo

Nicolás Fresedo and his wife Clotilde García were productive parents. On 5 May 1897 they welcomed their eighth child in to the world: Osvaldo Nicolás Fresedo. Osvaldo was encouraged to learn music and started first of all on his mother's piano and then on his father's concertina, accompanying his older violinist brother Emilio. At the age of fifteen in 1912 he was excited about going to a café in the neighbouring barrio to hear a bandoneón. He thought about his parents' gramophone records that he listened to at home: *Don Juan* and *Hotel Victoria* by Vicente Greco and *El Apache Argentino* and *Emancipacion* by Juan Maglio. Both produced extraordinary music from the mysterious bandoneón. Was he being too hopeful by thinking that he would hear something similar by the visiting trio? He knew it would be a special evening for him but he could have had no idea that the impact of the experience would shape the rest of his life.

He recalled many years later that he was in a Palermo café and from his table he could see the musicians at the bar. Their instrument cases gave some clues: one was violin-shaped, the other a guitar, but the third gave no hint as to the instrument within - it was just a box. The musicians looked around the café. There were the usual assortment of disinterested customers getting on with their normal evenings; chatting, drinking, eating, playing cards. The musicians did not notice the 15-year-old boy who was only there because of them, or more specifically because of one of them. They took up their allocated positions: Domingo placed his guitar on his knee; Francisco his violin to his shoulder; and Augusto opened up the box and took out his bandoneón placing it across his lap. They began to tune up but young Osvaldo had eyes only for Augusto's fingers on the buttons and the breathing of the bandoneón. In that café the young musicians were guitarist Domingo Salerno, violinist Francisco Canaro, and bandoneonist Augusto Berto. The watching boy, Osvaldo Fresedo, grew in to one of the most significant and longest lasting tango maestros - playing and recording for the next 50 years. That evening Osvaldo Fresedo went home elated and soon bought a concertina to learn the keys and scales. He started to feel his way around the instrument and produced reasonable versions of his favourite tangos. Within a year, on 31 May 1913, he formed a quartet with his brother Emilio on violin and another two brothers (Pedro and Martín Barreto) on guitars. Later that year he was on stage in a cabaret club playing the bandoneón in a short scene being enacted from the play *Una noche de garufa*.

In 1916 he was the bandoneonist at the Cabaret Montmartre in the quintet of José Martínez (piano), Francisco Canaro and Rafael Rinaldi (violins), and Leopoldo Thompson (double-bass). By then he was firmly amongst the leading tango musicians in the city. In 1916 he was in the much expanded orchestra playing for the carnival crowd at the Teatro Politeama in the city of Rosario. He was with:

- bandoneonists Vicente Greco, Juan Labissier and Pedro Polito;
- violinists Francisco and Rafael Canaro;
- pianists Samuel Castriota and José Martinez;
- double bassist Leopoldo Thompson; and
- the woodwind was provided by flautist Vicente Pecci and clarinetist Juan Carlos Bazán.

Osvaldo had similarly come to the attention of Roberto Firpo who in 1916 recorded one of Osvaldo's first tango compositions *El espiante*[104]. The following year at the Rosario carnival he was in the all-star line-up of the supersized Firpo-Canaro orchestra, sitting alongside bandoneonists Eduardo Arolas, Juan Deambroggio, Minotto Di Cicco, and Pedro Polito.

In April 1917, back in Buenos Aires, a couple of Victor sound engineers (George Cheney & Charles Althouse) had arrived from New York with portable recording equipment in order to capture tango music in Buenos Aires. In particular they had been sent to locate bandoneonist Vicente Loduca who had recorded in New York back in 1914[105]. Loduca did not have an orchestra at that time and so headed for the cabaret Royal Pigalle where a ready-made

---

[104] that Fresedo went on to record in 1927, 1932, 1933, 1955, and 1979
[105] see *Loduca* section below

quintet was playing: Osvaldo Fresedo (bandoneón), Julio Doutry and Francisco Canaro (violins), José Martínez (piano), and Leopoldo Thompson (double bass). The subsequent Victor recording was advertised as the Loduca-Fresedo orchestra and noted (as an extra attraction) that there were two bandoneóns. In a later interview Fresedo was asked whether he and Loduca interplayed with 'two voices[106]' but he dispelled any notion of creative innovation by saying that they just played anything because the Victor engineers didn't know any better. Nevertheless this was an orchestra of considerable talent with musicians who were about to shape and influence the tango dance music with which we are now so familiar in 21st century milongas. Shortly afterwards Fresedo's relationship with Canaro soured and he left (and was subsequently replaced by Canaro's brother Juan). He then joined up with pianist Juan Carlos Cobián and violinist Tito Rocatagliata. Cobián and Fresedo had much in common at both a personal and professional level. Both were more socially sophisticated than the average tango musician and their musical interpretation equally refined. Together they experimented with more complex musical arrangements, interweaving counter melodies and individual expression, and their audiences loved it. They remained together until the end of 1918 during which time Fresedo's name had started to appear in newspapers as a tango composer[107].

On 1 July 1919 Fresedo presented his first sextet at the Casino Pigalle in Buenos Aires consisting of pianist José María Rizzuti whose style perfectly matched that of Cobián, his second bandoneón was Pedro Maffia, and second violinist Julio De Caro.

---

[106] Meaning had the bandoneons played a sophisticated melody and counter-melody

[107] Examples include the now little known *Amionoco, Meneguina, El comisionado*

A new and popular style of complex, more thoughtful tango was emerging that in years to come would be almost exclusively (and unfairly) assigned to the name of De Caro. Whilst the sextet was in full flow Fresedo was offered a contract to travel to the Victor recording studios in the USA to form a new tango orchestra - the Orquesta Típica Select. Fresedo informed his musicians that he was leaving but that the sextet should continue to play. He introduced his long standing friend, bandoneonist Pedro Polito, as the new leader to replace him much to their surprise (and a few personal disappointments).

Fresedo then set sail on his new adventure to New York with pianist Enrique Delfino and violinist Tito Roccatagliata.

Vicente Greco

Vicente Greco had no idea that he would be securing his place in tango history when (from December 1909 to February 1910) he was invited by the retailer Casa Tagini to make recordings on the Columbia label. He went to the temporary recording room with his guitarist brother Domingo, and flautist 'El Tano' Vicente Pecci[108]. The two visiting engineers, William Freiburg and Gus Forbush, made at least 22 masters (18 tangos, 2 vals, and 2 polkas) and shipped them to Connecticut, North America for the manufacture of the records, that arrived in Argentina in May 1910. The first records went on sale in July 1910 and the advertisement in the magazine *Caras y Caretas* declared new tangos by an Orquesta Especial Típica Criolla. It did not name Greco and unfortunately for

GRANDES NOVEDADES

en Discos Columbia de $ 2.50

Selecto repertorio de todos los tangos criollos nuevos ejecutados por una orquesta especial típica criolla.

Discos Odeón COLUMBIA
y Fonotipia de Celebridades
VENTAS POR MAYOR Y MENOR

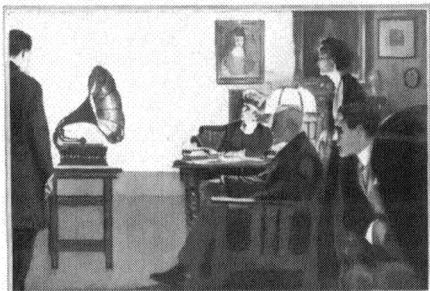

Un Grafófono **Columbia** hace las delicias del hogar y equivale á escuchar en casa conciertos musicales de mérito extraordinario. Es insustituible para las veladas familiares y fiestas íntimas.

him the record labels were misspelt as 'Orquesta Grego Orquesta Tipica Criolla' but his correct name would soon become a

---

[108] Some say that on some recordings there was also a violin but after several hours of listening I have decided to remain neutral on that point

household name. His recordings were the first to be described as (what would in due course be reduced to) an 'Orquesta Típica' in relation to this style of tango group. Vicente Greco therefore has the historic honour of forming, directing, and recording tango's first Orquesta Típica. The creation of such a name is likely to have been Casa Tagini's marketing idea to differentiate their style of tango from other tango offerings. Up to that point tango recordings had been comic songs, piano solos, string ensembles, and brass bands and so this was not only 'Criolla' but it was also decidedly 'Especial' and was centred around the new instrument of the bandoneón. An orquesta típica did not indicate exclusive dedication to tangos (as many later commentators tend to assert) but only that the group included a bandoneón. Greco's first recordings were a tribute to the tango pianist Rosendo Mendizábal[109] appropriately entitled *Rosendo* and the already long-established *Don Juan* by Ernesto Ponzio. The other popular tangos included compositions still known today (thanks to recordings by later orchestras):

- *El incendio* composed by Arturo De Bassi;
- *Hotel Victoria* by Feliciano Latasa;
- *Joaquina* by Juan Bergamino; and
- *La c... de la l...* by Manual Campoamor[110].

Today we are accustomed to the myth that such unrefined music and musicians were shunned by refined society and so it may surprise us to see the accompanying drawing in that first advertisement (above) that reveals the intended market for the records. It shows a formally dressed upper-class family gathered together at home, staring intently at the gramophone horn,

---

[109] see *Get To Know the Tango Pioneers: Origins to 1909*
[110] the edited wording of this tango refers to its earlier crude title, see *Get To Know the Tango Pioneers Origins to 1909/Pianists/Campoamor*

listening to the recordings of a tango band from the arrabal with a sound featuring the bandoneón. Although the new tango scene was now underway these recordings did not lead to an immediate change in the public's tango-listening habits. The more familiar string ensembles (rondallas) and brass bands continued to record tangos and to sell extensively.

In 1912 Greco returned to the Casa Tagini and recorded 14 tangos as the Orquesta Típica Greco (the name shortened from 'orquesta especial típica criolla') with the labels identifying a V. Greco as the director. Despite the grand title of orquesta típica the musicians were simply a trio: bandoneón, guitar, and flute. That same trio was also invited to record in 1912 by Alfredo Améndola who had just established his Atlanta recording facilities. To create a difference with the Tagini/Columbia recordings Améndola added a fourth member (Samuel Castriota as guitarist/pianist) and labelled the quartet as a quintet - the Quinteto Criollo Garrote. 'Garrote' was Vicente Greco's nickname, a name confusingly shared with his older brother Fernando. They recorded 20 tangos including Greco's own compositions:

COMPOSITION	BEST KNOWN RECORDED VERSIONS
El estribo	Rodolfo Biagi (1940)
Estoy penando	Roberto Firpo (1938, 1950)

In 1913/14 Greco again recorded as the Quintet Criollo Garrote but this time with an added violinist, Francisco Canaro. The 22 recordings included 7 compositions by Greco and 12 by Canaro - a sign of Canaro's ascendency and growing assertiveness. In 1914, to celebrate their income from the record sales, Greco and Canaro treated themselves to a beach holiday together in Montevideo. In his autobiography Canaro included a photograph of the two of them on the Playa de los Pocitos in striped swimwear at the foot of a bathing hut.

In the years 1910 to 1916 Greco's orquesta típica was sometimes a trio, a quartet, a quintet, and other times a sextet. The latter consisted of Vicente Greco and Juan Labissier on bandoneóns, Domingo Greco on piano, Francisco Canaro and Juan Abate on violins, and 'El Tano' Vicente Pecci on flute. They played at the Café Eden in La Boca, the Café El Estribo in San Cristóbal, and the dance hall San Martín on the street of Rodríguez Peña in the centre of the city. One Saturday night in 1911 Greco played his new tango, the rapid tempo *Rodríguez Peña,* and the assembled

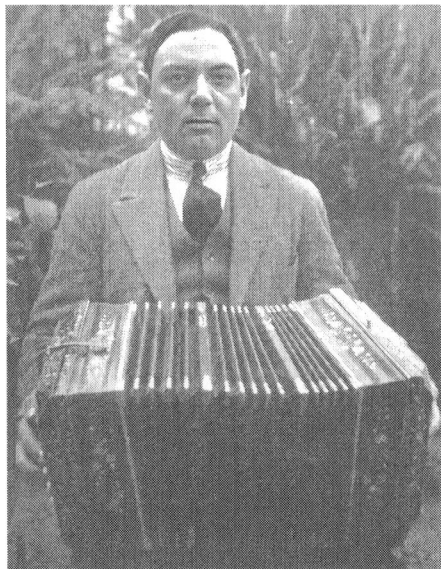

dancers went wild, lifting him on to their shoulders and parading him out in to the street (or so the story goes). Such was its popularity that Juan Maglio recorded it the following year (1912) and Genaro Espósito in 1914 but today we know it best from the versions by Francisco Canaro (1927, 1938, 1953 and 1959), Orquesta Típica Victor (1927), Juan D'Arienzo (1938), Osvaldo Fresedo (1927, 1942), and Carlos Di Sarli (1945, 1952, 1956) and many other artists.

In February and March 1914 the Greco sextet performed at the annual carnival celebrations in the Teatro Nacional. During the rest of the year and in 1915 Greco became the darling of the upper-classes and played at the great hotels and residences of the city. Such was Greco's status that on 29 October 1915 the Buenos Aires magazine *Fray Mocho* published a three-page article on him together with his brothers Domingo and Ángel, sister Elena, and mother María. That fact alone is extraordinary because no other artist, tango or otherwise, had received such extensive coverage up to that point. Despite today's myths and misunderstandings it is abundantly clear that the enjoyment of tango music from the arrabal was never restricted to the underclass of the city. Greco and his musicians played in the grand Plaza Hotel and the homes of the rich and famous for an enviable 200 pesos for each performance. The market for Greco's music sheets was mainly the musically trained, piano-owning middle and upper class families in Buenos Aires. Greco said that by October 1915 his most successful music sheet sales to date had been his tango compositions *El morochito* (22,000 copies), *Rodríguez Peña* (12,000), and in the first three months of being on sale his tango *El flete* had sold 6,000 copies.

Amongst Grecos many tango compositions are those that are still familiar to today's tango fans due to the recordings by later orchestras, for example:

COMPOSITION	BRST KNOWN RECORDED VERSIONS
Barba de choclo	Carlos Di Sarli (1945, 1952)
El estribo	Rodolfo Biagi (1940)
El flete	Juan D'Arienzo (1936), Francisco Canaro (1939)
El morochito	Enrique Rodríguez (1941)

El pibe	Orquesta Típica Victor (1933)
Estoy penando	Roberto Firpo (1938, 1950)
La viruta	Juan D'Arienzo (1936), Francisco Canaro (1938), Rodolfo Biagi (1948), and Carlos Di Sarli (1943 and 1952)
Ojos negros	Francisco Lomuto (1927), Osvaldo Fresedo (1927), Francisco Canaro (1932, 1949), Roberto Firpo (1937, 1942), Carlos Di Sarli (1945), Aníbal Troilo (1948), Juan D'Arienzo (1969)
Pof pof	Juan D'Arienzo (1948)
Racing Club (described as a Tango Futbalistico and dedicated to the football club of that name)	Carlos Di Sarli (1930, 1940), Aníbal Troilo (1940), Ángel D'Agostino (1946), Alfredo Gobbi Junior (1949), Rodolfo Biagi (1950)
Rodríguez Peña	Osvaldo Fresedo (1927, 1942), Francisco Canaro (1927, 1938, 1953), Julio De Caro (1930), Roberto Firpo (1937), Juan D'Arienzo (1938,1966), Carlos Di Sarli (1945, 1952, 1956)

I am surprised, and saddened, that more of his compositions were not amongst the repertoire of the later dance orchestras whose recordings still fill today's milongas around the world. However we can listen[111] to some of Greco's other compositions that did not make it beyond his own recordings, for example:

Pachequito, Los muchachos, Chochita, Que queres?, El garrotazo, Pulmonia doble, Don Pedrito (co-written with his brother Domingo) and *Vicentito* (co-written with Agustín Bardi). The latter ends with

---

[111] on the website of Discography of American Historical Recordings (DAHR)

the suggestion of what later became the trademark ending of tangos, known as the 'chan chan'.

It is interesting to track down the original published sheet music of tangos as many have personal dedications from the composer (although the context and relevance of many are now often obscure). Vicente had a tendency to dedicate his compositions to friends, sponsors, and pleasingly his fellow tango pioneers:

- *El perverso* is dedicated, intriguingly, to Roberto Firpo. The drawing on the sheet music shows a pianist attacking his piano with his piano stool - there is obviously a back story here waiting to be discovered;
- *Tiene la palabra* is dedicated to Francisco Lomuto in his role as the Secretary to the Sociedad Nacional de Autores Compositores y Editores de Música, as well as a friend and colleague;
- *De raza* is dedicated to the pianist Pascual Cardarópoli (who played in the trios and quartets of Eduardo Arolas, Roberto Firpo, and Pedro Maffia) and violinist Domingo Petillo (who played in 1916 with Pedro Maffia and Francisco Lomuto); and
- *Los soñadores* (The Dreamers) is dedicated to his pianist friends Enrique Delfino, Juan Carlos Cobían, and Carlos Geroni Flores. One can only speculate why Greco linked them with that title but I suspect it was because of their romantic style of compositions (known as tango romanza).

By 1919 Greco was a successful tango composer and performer. He was 31 years old (younger than Roberto Firpo and the same age as Francisco Canaro) and seemingly on track to establish himself further as a leading figure in the coming decades.

Unfortunately he was living with an injury, sustained whilst performing on a raised gallery that collapsed. This resulted in a nasty fall and internal injuries to his lungs and kidneys. The injury affected his walk to such an extent that he needed a stick to support himself. The titles of two of his tangos appear to reference those difficulties in his life: *El garrotazo* (a huge physical blow) and *Pulmonia doble* (double pneumonia, an affliction of the lungs). Nevertheless Greco continued to perform, mainly at dance halls, until 1921 when he became increasingly unwell. Just before midnight on 5 October 1924, at the age of 36, he died from kidney failure. We can never know what enduring recording legacy Vicente Greco may have created had he survived to the period of the more advanced electric recording era that was introduced a year later in 1925.

Vicente Loduca

Saverio Loduca, his wife Miquela, and their young son Vicente emigrated from Italy to Argentina in the 1890s and set up home in a town north of Buenos Aires. Young Vicente studied music, married, and then moved to the barrio of La Boca in Buenos Aires where he played his bandoneón at local cafés. One of them was the Café Royal where in 1908 he led a trio with violinist Francisco Canaro and pianist Samuel Castriota. He became a regular and admired tango performer and teacher of the bandoneón, being one of the very few that could read music notation. In August 1911 he advertised his services in the music magazine *El Gaucho Relampago,* offering bandoneón lessons and providing orchestras[112] for dance halls and café-bars.

---

[112] 'orchestra' at that time meant anything from a trio up to a sextet

In 1913 he formed a quartet with Celestino Ferrer on piano, and both José Sentio and Eduardo Monelos on violin. They became the regular band at a café on the street of Entre Ríos, in the basement of which was a tango dance academy 'Cain y Abel'. In April that year the journalist, Luis Sixto Clara, visited the dance class in order to write an article entitled 'El Tango' for the magazine *Sherlock Holmes*. His purpose was to interview the director Casimiro Ain but as he

Vicente Lo Duca

Da leciones de Bandonión, organiza orquesta para Baile y Bares

CONSTITUCION 2140

walked through the café he was struck by the music of the 'well-known and popular' quartet. It was the first time that he had heard a bandoneón and he described its sound as seductive, sad and that it had something 'of ourselves, of our character, something of the spirit of the jota[113]'. He wrote that the music stirred emotions in his heart and soul that he could not describe other than as a deep sense of nostalgia, 'a sad happiness, a joyful sadness.' During the interview Casimiro Ain[114] invited him to visit again the following day in order to hear a concert of bandoneóns. When he returned he met and interviewed Vicente Loduca. Also there were bandoneonists Augusto Berto and Domingo Santa Cruz. Loduca explained the unfamiliar instrument to the journalist, starting quite practically by saying that it originated in Germany arriving over 30 years ago as a crude instrument that had some design similarities to the accordion but the sound was as different as day and night. He said that the new instrument had found its way to the dimly lit dance halls but was certainly not welcome at first in the refined

---

[113] a traditional Spanish musical genre
[114] see *Dancers* section above

salons and as a result few wanted to learn how to play it. Within a couple of minutes Vicente Loduca's passion for the instrument and for tango music opened up: 'if you can hear…if you know how to feel…if you have a soul…if you have loved…if you have a lover…there is nothing more sentimental…nothing that gets to the depths of your soul…that lifts you to the unimaginable heights of infinity'. Although he appeared to have made his point convincingly he nevertheless continued 'Believe me the bandoneón is…have you ever been alone on a rainy night and heard the mysterious purring of a cat…have you ever been in bed on one of those cold, freezing nights, nestled in the blankets worrying about an unknown future knowing that you are alone and you hear the distant notes of a neighbour's piano that seem to slip away in to the far off night but you would like to capture them and make them yours'. And so he continued by conjuring up images of a howling dog and a pale moon as one's only companion, watching dancing couples through a window and he concluded 'all of that in one note of the bandoneón'. Loduca said that the journey of the bandoneón was similar to that of the guitar but in reverse. More than 50 years earlier (being the 1850s to 1860s) the guitar had been a respected instrument, even amongst the aristocracy, and represented the proud legends of the gauchos and the pampas but 'today the gaucho has disappeared, the guitar has been replaced by the piano and the violin, and the guitar is only played now in the lowest of venues…whereas years ago people were embarrassed by the bandoneón but today it has arrived…as there are many playing it from the arrabal to the city centre, even in the Avenida de Mayo, and that many passing pedestrians stop at cafés to hear its distinct sounds'. Remember that this interview was in April 1913, making it a contemporary and authoritative account that tango played on bandoneón was already popular across the city and across the social classes.

Meanwhile the bandoneón concert had begun and the journalist agreed with what Loduca had said, that the sound indeed 'had much of the guitar, of the pampas, of the vidalita[115]'. Frustratingly, he did not publish any conversations he may have had with Augusto Berto nor Domingo Santa Cruz although his companion did take each of them out in to the tiny courtyard for a portrait photograph[116]. Loduca also told the journalist that he and his musicians were about to travel imminently with Casimiro Ain to Paris. They had a contract there to record with Pathé and they would also jointly open a dance academy to teach the Parisians how to dance tango properly.

For some reason the violinist José Sentio was unable to travel with them and so the five young tango hopefuls (Loduca, Ferrer, Monelos, Ain and his wife Marta) boarded the steamship *Sierra Ventana* and sailed from Buenos Aires to Europe. Vicente Loduca was the first Argentinian tango bandoneonist to travel to Europe and, soon after his arrival, Pathé recorded his bandoneón solo *El Argentino*. The trio recorded another 57 tracks labelled variously as Orquesta Típica Vicente Loduca, Orquesta Loduca, and the Rondalla Ferrer conducted by Loduca. The Pathé outlet in Buenos Aires, on the central Avenida de Mayo, advertised the 'brand new repertoire by

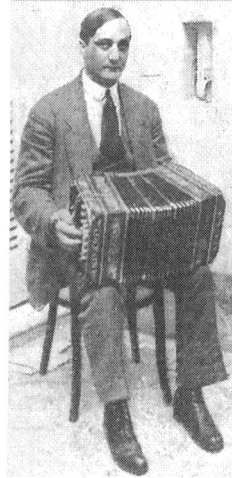

---

[115] a folk genre from the northern provinces of Argentina
[116] the photographs of Berto and Santa Cruz from that day appear in their respective sections of this chapter

the most famous orquesta típica criolla Loduca, Ferrer y Monelos'. The publicity included a photograph (taken prior to the French trip) that misleadingly included José Senito who was not on the recordings. Their recordings of the popular tangos of the day included many that are still regularly heard due to the versions by later orchestras: *Una noche de garufa*, *Rodríguez Peña*, *Un copetin*, *El caburé*, *Argañaráz*, *El tamango*, *El irresistible*, *Sentimiento criollo* and the valses *Francia* and *Pabellón de las Rósas*.

Amongst one of their enthralled admirers in Paris was a wealthy American lady who funded them to travel to New York. The US immigration records at Ellis Island show Vicente Loduca, Celestino Ferrer, Eduardo Monelos, Casimiro and Marta Ain arriving in 1913 on board a ship from Le Havre, France. In New York they performed for high society, Casimiro and Marta Ain opened a tango dance academy, and the trio recorded for the Victor Talking Machine Company that needed a genuine Argentinian orquesta típica to compete with the widely successful Roberto Firpo on Odeon. The Victor company was in no doubt about the intended market and it was not in the USA: the ledgers were marked 'For Export' and destined for Argentina. On 7 January 1914, under the name Orquesta Argentina Loduca, the trio recorded 7 double-sided discs including the compositions of Rosendo Mendizábal *El entrerriano*, Alfredo Bevilacqua's *Independencia*, and Vicente Greco's *La viruta*, plus several of their own compositions. In November 1914 Victor advertisements in Buenos Aires showed tangos by the 'Orquesta Criolla Loduca (Bandoleón)' and the following November (1915) the same recordings were advertised as by the 'Orquesta Típica Argentina, con Bandoleón, de V. Loduca'. The misspelling of the instrument was quite common even amongst the experts in the music industry. The advertisement itself included a photograph of the trio together with Casimiro and Marta Ain dancing alongside them

---

The violinist Eduardo Monelos left the USA and returned home to Argentina where he played in the trios of bandoneonist Graciano De Leone in Buenos Aires and of Genaro Espósito in Córdoba. At only 24 years of age he was on track to become a successful tango musician over the coming decades (and in to the era of recordings that still fill the dance halls of today). He was younger than his peers Francisco Canaro and Osvaldo Fresedo, he had the necessary tango talent, and had accrued experience of the international music business. Nobody could have expected that he would be dead before his 26th birthday, struck down by tuberculosis in 1917.

In 1917 the Victor Talking Machine Company wanted to revive its offering of tango recordings with the successful Vicente Loduca and Celestino Ferrer orchestra. On 3 March 1917 the Victor engineers George Cheney and the fluent Spanish-speaking Charles Althouse boarded the *S.S Tennyson* bound for Buenos Aires together with their portable recording equipment. Memories differ about who it was that they met first and who asked whom to form an orchestra but the summary is that Loduca did not have a group of musicians but he did know the quintet of Canaro and Martínez performing at the cabaret Royal Pigalle. Together they presented themselves to Cheney & Althouse as the Orquesta Típica Loduca with Osvaldo Fresedo as second bandoneón, violinists Francisco Canaro and Julio Doutry, pianist José Martínez, double bassist Leopoldo Thompson, and a flautist. On their first day in the makeshift studio, 30 April 1917, the engineers took a while to arrange the positioning of the instruments in order to achieve a balanced recording. In the Victor ledger one of them noted 'For Take 1, double bass at rear of room; for Take 2 double bass out'.

But after listening to Take 2 he noted that some of the musicians had made a 'complaint about the weak flute' but further enquiry 'revealed Loduca had instructed the fluter to play very softly'. The septet returned on 2 May and Leopoldo Thompson was still relegated to the back of the room to reduce his heavy bass notes that were distorting the combined sound. They made two recordings that day but when they returned on the 4 May their next 15 recordings were entirely without Thompson and his double bass.

Unfortunately many of their chosen tangos are no longer heard today but those that are still familiar were:

TITLE	BEST KNOWN RECORDED VERSIONS
La huella	Roberto Firpo (1939), Ricardo Tanturi (1941), Rodolfo Biagi (1946)
Lagrimas y sonrisas	Juan D'Arienzo (1936), Rodolfo Biagi (1941)
Peñas de amor	Juan D'Arienzo (1935)
Cara sucia	Francisco Canaro (1937), Carlos Di Sarli (1942, 1952, 1957)

In 1917 and 1918 they recorded 28 tangos as the Orquesta Típica Loduca with the label stressing the 'two bandoneons Loduca-Fresedo'. I suspect that Canaro felt aggrieved that his name was not in the top line because by late 1918 he had managed to restyle the group to become known (on some occasions) by the twin title 'Loduca-Canaro'.

Vicente Loduca is little known today. The recordings he made between 1915 and 1918 are too early to be played at milongas (due to their preserved sound quality) and his few compositions were not recorded by the later orchestras. We can remember him therefore for the role he played establishing and promoting the bandoneón in the first decade of the 1900s and for being the named orchestra leader who increased the recording profiles of the future leaders and recording stars Francisco Canaro and Osvaldo Fresedo.

Pedro Maffia

In early 1918 in a suburb of Bahía Blanca Carlos Gardel, José Razzano and their guitarist José Ricardo were on tour together with the tango quintet of Roberto Firpo. Having a free evening José Ricardo went out to listen to another band of musicians and was impressed by the bandoneón player, so much so that he reported back to Firpo and his bandoneonist Juan Deambroggio. They in turn went to check out this unknown bandoneonist and were taken by his distinctive style of seated stillness, gently teasing out the notes by only partly opening and closing the bellows. They recruited him, thereby creating a sextet (pianist Firpo, bandoneonists Deamboggio and Maffia, violinists Agesilao Ferrazzano and Cayetano Puglisi, and a flautist). Despite his youthful 18 years the calm presence and playing style of Pedro Maffia improved the maturity of their overall sound.

In late 1919 Maffia had grown tired after months of touring with Firpo and when the group was in Córdoba he decided to leave, without any alternative plan. Firpo had to quickly find a replacement and a local 15-year-old bandoneonist was highly recommended to him. Maffia's sudden departure opened up an opportunity for Ciríaco Ortiz who proved to be a valuable find, replacement, and core tango virtuoso in the coming decades[117].

Back in Buenos Aires, Maffia linked up with violinist Julio De Caro and pianist José María Rizutti who had similarly split from their orchestra leader, in their case Eduardo Arolas. The three of them worked well together and established a rapport that would lead them to collaborate again in later years. Soon afterwards De Caro and Rizutti joined the sextet of Osvaldo Fresedo who had a contract at the Casino Pigall whereas Maffia after a short spell with Fresedo was sweet-talked back to Firpo by the affable Leopoldo Thompson. Maffia returned frequently to the line-up of Roberto Firpo and appeared on many of his recordings up to 1928.

In the 1920s Maffia went on to shape the sound of another sextet that, regardless of his protestations, became known as the Orquesta Típica Julio De Caro. Despite Maffia's significant musical influence the orchestra's style of tango music became known as Decarean (from the orchestra's leader De Caro[118]).

---

[117] see *Get To Know the Tango Pioneers 1920 to 1935*
[118] see *Violinists/De Caro* below

Juan Maglio

Juan Maglio had been performing across the city of Buenos Aires, and its surrounding provinces, since 1899[119]. In 1912 Maglio's quartet was touring the café venues of Buenos Aires. Maglio sat in the centre with his bandoneón across his lap; standing on each side were José Pepino Bonano playing the violin with a cornet attachment (much like the one that was made famous by Julio De Caro some 15 years later); Carlos Hernani Macchi was playing the flute; and Luciano Ríos with his seven-stringed guitar was providing bass and a percussive swing rhythm, the pre-cursor to the tango double-bass. One of the other regular venues for Maglio was La Paloma in Palermo - an inexplicably popular café for the locals who were not at all deterred by the nightly fights nor by the rats that ran amok between the tables. This was not a venue for dancing and yet tango dancers

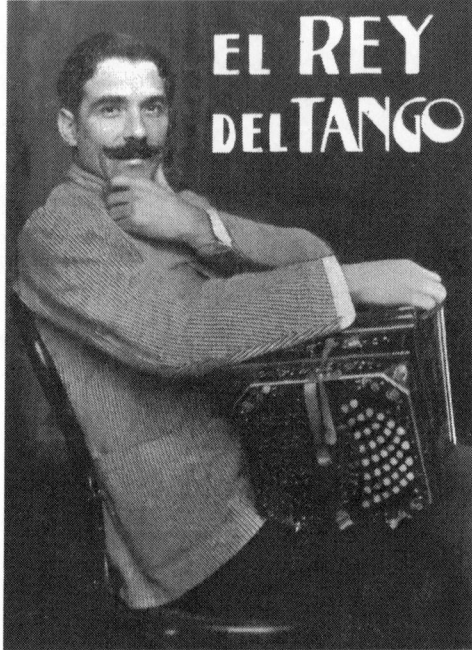

EL REY DEL TANGO

---

[119] see *Get To Know the Tango Pioneers Origins to 1909*

such as El Cachafaz[120] came to listen to their music. It was at La Paloma that representatives of the Casa Tagini[121] came to assess Maglio and offered him a recording contract that launched him to superstar status after more than a decade of established popularity as a tango musician.

Juan Maglio holds the historic position of being the first to record a solo on the bandoneón - the tango *La sonambula* (1912). His recordings were labelled as Orquesta Típica Pacho with director J. Maglio, although the orchestra was in fact a quartet (with Luciano Ríos having been replaced by a guitarist with a similar style, Leopoldo Thompson). In 1913 Casa Tagini/Columbia further elevated Maglio's status by giving him his own distinctive label bearing not only his name but his photograph and signature. On 24 February 1913 the 'famous teacher of the Bandoleón Juan Maglio Pacho' wrote to José Tagini saying that all of his friends and all of those who appreciated his music knew that neither he nor his orchestra had played on any record except those produced by Casa Tagini. He wrote that he was declaring this so that no unscrupulous businessman could wrongly use his name, or his nickname 'Pacho', to misrepresent recordings that he had granted exclusively to Tagini. The letter may throw light on another tango misunderstanding: many repeated accounts say that Maglio was so popular that customers at record stores would simply ask for a 'Pacho' when buying a tango record. The understanding is that customers knew that the artist was not Maglio and simply used the word Pacho as a generic term for a tango record. Maglio and

---

[120] see Dancers section above
[121] a music retailer, publisher, and exclusive agent and recording house for the Columbia Phonograph Company

Tagini were clear in their message that tango records were being fraudulently labelled as Pacho in order to deceive the public.

Maglio's fame and fortunes increased rapidly. He and his quartet were never without work although Maglio himself did not always make the effort to turn up at the venues. For example in 1913, whilst contracted at the Café Gariboto, he frequently disappeared for a few days with his latest passing lover and relied on his emergency stand-in, Manuel Pizarro, to play the bandoneón in his place.

In 1915 the magazine *Fray Mocho* published a two-page article on Juan Maglio entitled 'El Rey del Tango' (The King of Tango) that included some excellent photographs: Maglio at four years of age, Maglio standing at the door to his house together with his wife - she in everyday clothing and he in tuxedo and bow tie, the pensive Maglio sitting with bandoneón on knee (above), and Maglio at home dressed casually studying music together with his formally dressed pianist Luis Suárez Tapia (below). The article explained that he had learnt the bandoneón first from his father and then from Domingo Santa Cruz (see below). He proudly described his first bandoneón as having 35 keys whereas his current (1915) bandoneón had 75. Maglio was not at all reluctant to talk about income saying that he went from performing at La Paloma where

he was paid 3 pesos a night, then gradually moved to the city centre when he started to earn 550 pesos a month, and then following his recording contracts in the year 1914/1915 he earned 12,000 pesos. He used some of that money to buy a café bar - called Ambos Mundos but

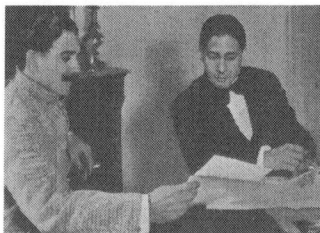

predictably known as Café Pacho - with his pianist Luis Suárez as co-owner plus a substantial investment by the music company Casa Tagini. Suddenly his fortunes changed for the worse After his recording successes in 1912 and 1913 he made no further recordings for another 8 years or more. That extremely long gap did not reflect a fall in his popularity but was due to the economic effect of the World War. Casa Tagini, in which he was a substantial investor, relied on its record production across the Atlantic in Europe[122]. Maglio started to lose a lot of money, in income and devalued capital investments, and at the same time his café also began to fall in to debt. Fortunately his music saved him - he continued to be in demand on both sides of the Río de la Plata, he had expanded his audiences to the homes of the rich and famous, to carnivals at prestigious venues such as the Pabellón de las Rosas, and to the theatre.

In 1917 he was once again in front of the recording horns. This time those set up by the visiting engineers George Cheney and Charles Althouse from the Victor Talking Machine Company. Between 24 and 27 April the quartet of bandoneonist Maglio, pianist Luis Suárez, flautist Carlos Macchi, and violinist José Bonano recorded 22 tracks. The Victor ledger entries routinely comprise factual data on who, what, and when but on occasions the sound engineer was moved to add a personal comment. Against the valses recorded on 25 April (*Recordar es vivir, Siempre tuyo, and Orillas del Plata*) he simply wrote 'Pretty valses'. On 27 April the quartet recorded *La paisana* and *Anda pato* for which Luis Suárez moved from the piano to the guitar and then returned to the piano stool, the engineer noting 'Guitar out and piano in'. They may only

---

[122] other companies such as Nacional Odeon rapidly made alternative production arrangements in Brazil

be five words but they help us to imagine the scene, with movement and discussions as well as the end product sound. It is clear that the engineers' technical decisions dictated the instruments and thereby how the musicians would be heard (and judged) by the listening public for generations to come.

Maglio continued to shape the tango sound in the following decade, recruiting (at different times) the young pianists Rodolfo Biagi and Ángel D'Agostino, bandoneonist Aníbal Troilo, violinist Elvino Vardaro and others. He recorded tangos until 1932 and (some of) the later ones are thankfully still heard and enjoyed at today's milongas.

Domingo Santa Cruz

Domingo Santa Cruz had been performing, mainly with his guitarist brother Juan, in the cafés and dance rooms of Buenos Aires since at least 1899. In 1904 he published his tango composition *Unión Cívica*, best known today by the recordings of Juan D'Arienzo (1938), Rodolfo Biagi (1938), and Osvaldo Pugliese (1958).

On Wednesday 21 September 1910 he walked in to a musical instrument shop and bought a new bandoneón with 71 buttons (38 providing the treble, 33 the bass) and paid 180 pesos. The 71 'voice' was the largest, the best, and the one that most bandoneón players in Buenos Aires aspired to own. In 1910 Domingo Santa Cruz was a successful bandoneonist and deserved the best.

In 1913 Vicente Loduca described Domingo Santa Cruz as the best bandoneonist that he knew. That was substantial praise as Loduca knew all of the big name players such as Arolas, Berto, Greco, and Maglio. In 1915 the newspaper *Crítica* added firther praise by saying that Domingo Santa Cruz was the leading representative of the 'plebeian bellows'. Yet despite his unchallenged status amongst tango musicians there is little known about him today because there are few surviving (or, at least, few discovered) documents about his life.

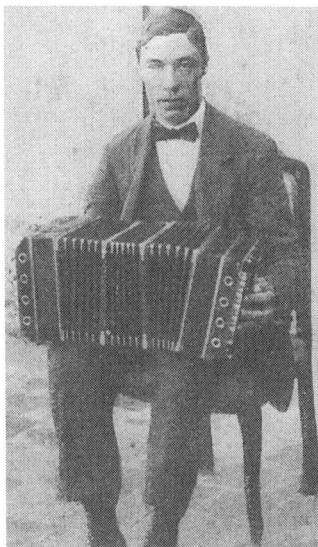

As well as being outstanding tango musicians Domingo and his brother Juan (by then a pianist) were also well-respected tango dance instructors. They had their own studio, between the barrios of Abasto and Alto Palermo, and were often invited in to the homes of wealthy clients to give private lessons. In July 1914 the brothers organised a three-day tango dance competition at their studios and offered the alluring prize of a man's tailor-made suit. They played their music for the dancers and tantalisingly promised a repertoire of new tangos although we no longer know which ones.

There is evidence that Domingo Santa Cruz continued to perform throughout this decade and the next, for example:

- in 1916 he was on tour in Montevideo with second bandoneonist Manuel Firpo (the bandoneón teacher of young Osvaldo Fresedo) and guitarist Luciano Ríos[123];
- in 1919 in Buenos Aires he was leading another trio, with guitarist Félix Camerano and young violinist Juan Pecci[124];
- in the 1920s he continued to play tangos on both sides of the Río de la Plata and broadcast on Radio Nacional and Radio Cultura.

In the late 1920s Domingo Santa Cruz became ill with tuberculosis. On 19 July 1931 the newspaper *Última Hora* grieved for the state of his health and during his final days the most famous tango stars held a benefit concert as a tribute to this great pioneer. Performing free of charge during a week-long vigil the musicians included the orchestras of Francisco Canaro, Julio De Caro, Francisco Lomuto, Edgardo Donato, Juan Maglio and Ricardo Brignolo; the singers included Ignacio Corsini, sisters Ada and Adhelma Falcón, and many more. The fact that the tango maestros that we admire today held him in such high regard is a reminder that we too should remember him, with gratitude for the music and dance that we enjoy so much today (even though he did not leave us any recordings and only a few compositions).

---

[123] up to that point also the regular guitarist with Juan Maglio
[124] son of the pioneer flautist Vicente and taught by Ernesto Ponzio

Others

In 1914 Roberto Firpo, Genaro Espósito, and Eduardo Arolas recorded Firpo's composition *Curda Completa* for which Firpo later published the sheet music together with his dedication to a long list of bandoneón players. He named 56 of them and further credited 'the others'. The list speaks volumes about the role of the bandoneonist and the esteem in which they were held. Those listed that have their own sections in the *Get To Know the Tango Pioneers* series were Eduardo Arolas, Arturo Bernstein, Augusto Berto, Genaro Espósito, Vicente Greco, Vicente Loduca, Juan 'Pacho' Maglio, Manuel Pizarro, Sebastián Ramos Mejía, and Domingo Santa Cruz.

Others on the list included:

- Juan Lorenzo Labissier, born in 1887, who was the second bandoneonist to Vincent Greco, Eduardo Arolas, Genaro Espósito, Arturo Bernstein, Domingo Santa Cruz and many more pioneering orchestra leaders. It is sometimes easy to overlook the musicians who did not become headline names yet it is clear that Juan Labissier was much admired, not only by tango fans but also by his peers. There are two tangos dedicated to him:
    - *Lorenzo* was composed by Agustín Bardi and is best known today by the recorded versions of Julio De Caro (1926), Osvaldo Fresedo (1927), Juan D'Arienzo (1936), Francisco Canaro (1927, 1938), and Osvaldo Pugliese (1965);
    - *El chamuyo* composed by Francisco Canaro and is today known by the recordings of Canaro himself (1927 & 1933), the Orquesta Típica Victor (1930), Edgardo Donato (1938), and Juan D'Arienzo (1965).

- Ricardo 'Mochila' González born in 1885 started as a tango guitarist (and taught the adolescent Eduardo Arolas how to play it) and like several others changed his instrument to the more fashionable bandoneón. He played with Greco, Canaro, and Berto, spent years playing in Paris and composed several tangos recorded by others including *La Rosarina* by Juan D'Arienzo (1937);

- Domingo Biggeri (right) was the leader of his own orquesta típica criolla and recorded on the Odeon label in 1914. His endorsement of satisfaction with Odeon appeared in an advertisement on 25 April in *Caras y Caretas* together with his photograph, alongside those of his peers Eduardo Arolas and Roberto Firpo;

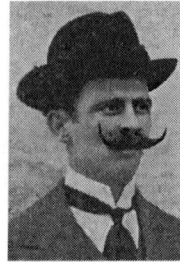

- Antonio Vicente Cacace, born in 1892 in Buenos Aires to Italian immigrant parents who taught him to play the mandolin. Having taken bandoneón lessons from Genaro Espósito by 1909 he became one of the many tango musicians playing in the lively Suarez and Necochea corner of La Boca. In 1926 he was selling and re-tuning bandoneons to support the still growing population of bandoneonists in Buenos Aires;

- Luis Solari who is remembered as the butcher who played in his local barrio with a bandoneón adorned with polished golden corners;

- Alfredo Fattini who learnt from another butcher named Domingo Cichitti and played with Natalín Felipetti who was described as already 'a very old bandoneonist';

- José Arturo Severino born in 1892, was taught by Sebastián Ramos Mejía and went on to teach others including in 1909 the young Juan Bautista Guido. Severino set up his own bandoneón school in 1911 and formed his own tango orchestra playing in theatres and cabarets. In March and April 1917 his orquesta típica (being a quartet of bandoneón, violin, flute and guitar) recorded 10 tracks that included his own composition *La bicoca*, that is best known today by the Juan D'Arienzo recording (1940);

- Antonio Chiappe in 1909 advertised himself in the newspapers as the best player of valses on the bandoneón and later led his own quintet.

5   Violinists

Canaro, D'Arienzo, De Caro, Ferrazzano, Puglisi, Rocatagliata

Francisco Canaro

Francisco Canaro had been performing tango as a violinist since

1906. Between 1910 and 1919 he established himself as a much sought-after performer, composer, orchestra leader, and recording star. He must have felt that by 1919, at the age of 29, he had reached the peak of his success.

Recordings
In 1913/14 the bandoneonist Vicente Greco recorded on

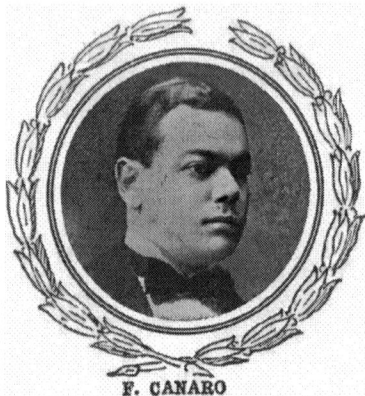

F. CANARO

the Atlanta label[125] and his violinist was Francisco Canaro. The discs were labelled not as an orquesta típica but as the Quinteto Criollo Garrote (which confusingly was a quartet). Their recordings included a dozen compositions by Canaro - a sign of his increasing talent and influence. Whilst there Canaro made an important professional connection with Atlanta's owner, Alfredo Améndola, who later that year invited Canaro back to record under his own name and to include his latest composition *El chamuyo*. Améndola, in accordance with his normal practice, shipped all of the master

---

[125] newly established by Alfredo Améndola

recordings to Germany where they were pressed in to discs with labels printed in Spanish and then sent back to Buenos Aires. Unfortunately, for everyone involved, the ship returning the crates of records was attacked and sunk. Améndola could no longer operate with his cross-Atlantic partners, but he did come up with an alternative plan. It involved Saverio Leonetti who had established a recording and disc manufacturing plant in Porto Alegre, Brazil. In 1915 Canaro was amongst the first Buenos Aires artists to benefit from those facilities.

Améndola could not afford to pay the cost of travel to Brazil of all of Canaro's quintet and so he took with him Canaro (violinist), Pedro Polito (bandoneonist), and Leopoldo Thompson (guitarist) and boarded the cargo ship *El Toro* bound for Porto Alegre, Brazil. They may have initially considered the coastal sea journey to have been safer than crossing the Atlantic to Europe but later changed their mind. For their return journey they opted to endure a three-day train journey. That proved to be a wise decision as their outbound ship, *El Toro*, was later sunk by a German submarine. Once at Porto Alegre, Saverio Leonetti (the owner of Casa A Electrica) and his recording technician, Francisco Schultz, hired a local violinist and flautist to form the required quintet. Canaro remembered the experience of recording there to have been physically uncomfortable due to most of the room's space being taken by the inordinately large receiving horns and the five musicians being cramped together. Nevertheless they did manage to record and were delighted with the quality of the discs produced. Canaro returned to Porto Alegre, Brazil in 1916, but with his own violinist Rafael Rinaldi, and again in 1917. Over the course of his three visits he recorded more than 70 of his most popular tunes (many of which are still familiar today in dance halls around the world, due to the recordings of orchestras in the 1930s to 1950s).

The recorded tangos included: *Charamusca, El flete, Didi, El espiante, Popoff, Nobleza gaucha, El amanecer, Royal Pigalle, El distinguido ciudadano, Germaine, Racing Club, La huella, Cara sucia, El moro, Rawson,* and *La polla* (that is known today as *Madreselva*); and the valses: *Aeroplano, Corazon de artistas, Pabellon de las Rosas, Lagrimas y sonrisas,* and *Vibraciones de alma.*

The discs were promoted in the Atlanta catalogue as part of the 'Canaro Series' in which Francisco Canaro was described as the popular 'national author' - a composer of national songs. The accompanying photograph showed a quintet that included pianist José Martínez (although he did not appear on the recordings). Tucked inside each printed copy of the Atlanta catalogue was an inserted slip of paper from Alfredo Améndola dated 9 August 1917: 'We are pleased to present to you our new list of recent arrivals whose perfect execution by the Orquesta Típica Canaro has justly awakened general admiration for being the only orchestra that has interpreted faithfully the true national feeling and aire.' Tango continued to be promoted as a national aire, a musical genre representing cultural pride.

In May 1917 Canaro recorded as one of the violinists in what was presented as the Orquesta Típica Vicente Loduca. The North American Victor Talking Machine Company had sent recording engineers George Cheney and Charles Althouse to Buenos Aires to record Argentinian artists. Victor had previously recorded bandoneonist Vicente Loduca (in 1915 in the USA) and part of the mission of Cheney and Althouse was to track him down. The result was that they found Loduca but, as he did not have an orchestra, he sought help from Canaro who did (a quintet of Canaro, Doutry, Fresedo, Martínez, and Thompson). The 'Loduca orchestra' presented to Cheney and Althouse therefore had two bandoneons that gave Victor an added novelty for their promotions. It must have been irritating for Canaro that not only was his orchestra being labelled as Loduca's but also marketed as Loduca-Fresedo. He managed to change that and in a Victor promotional advert on 28 September 1918 the name was changed to Orquesta Típica Loduca-Canaro. Although he still had to concede second place the advertisement did at least carry his photograph and not Loduca's. Canaro was a determined businessman. One of their recording days, Tuesday 15 May 1917, has a unique place in Victor Talking Machine's recording history. For the privilege of recording the tango *Cara sucia* (of which Canaro was noted as composer[126]) the orchestra (probably led by Canaro) demanded an extra payment. The demand and the amount was so unusual that the sound engineers Cheney & Althouse felt compelled to make a note in the ledger: 'Victor Talking Machine paid large price for privilege to record - paid to holder of artist's contract, (Alfredo) Améndola'. There is no other similar note in any of the other Victor ledger entries, for any other recording, by any other artist.

On 11 April 1918, the weekly illustrated Buenos Aires magazine *Atlántida* published the full music score of the tango *Cara sucia* under the article title 'What the people are singing' and it showed the arrangement and music by F. Canaro.

---

[126] Canaro arranged the tune but did not compose it. See *Get To Know the Tango Pioneers Origens to 1909*

<u>Performances</u>

Canaro was always working. In August 1911 he placed a small advertisement in the first edition of the music magazine *El Gaucho Relampago* aimed at those that wanted an orchestra[127] for dances or in bars. Francisco was already showing himself to be more than a casual musician for hire, he saw himself as an organiser and leader.

However like many musicians he would take work when he could. It was not unusual for musicians to play in several bands during the same period, sometimes as a supporting musician and other times as the nominal leader.

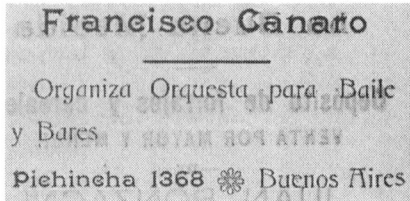

Francisco Canaro

Organiza Orquesta para Baile y Bares

Pichincha 1368 ❀ Buenos Aires

On 21 September 1914 Canaro provided the orchestra for the first 'Baile del Internado', which was the first day of spring celebration for the students of the prestigious Buenos Aires Faculty of Medicine. In terms of socio-economic positions the Faculty of Medicine and its members were amongst the highest professional classes and yet, in 1914, they chose to launch their first annual celebration not only with tango music but with a group from the arrabal[128]. The Bailes del Internado soon became infamous for their macabre pranks when students produced various body parts from the morgue during their celebrations until predictably the horror increased and the authorities stopped all further events. The tribute tango *El internado* was first recorded by Canaro in 1917 but the best-known versions today are by Canaro himself (1935), Juan D'Arienzo (1938), and Rodolfo Biagi (1953).

---

[127] at that time an orchestra was anything from a trio to a sextet
[128] more evidence to refute the myth of tango being rejected by the 'establishment' classes. See *Get To Know the Tango Pioneers Origins to 1909*.

Despite his established role as an orchestra leader Canaro was not above being a hired violinist for somebody else. In 1915 he played in the trio of bandoneonist Manuel Pizarro with guitarist 'El Negro' Ortiz. Pizarro recalled that, whilst playing, Canaro shook his head so much that he attracted the nickname of 'the cocktail shaker'. It is a pity that all of the film clips that we have of Canaro are from his more mature days sedately conducting his orchestra. That year Canaro played in more than one band, in more than one venue, often in the same evening finishing one at midnight then racing off to start another session elsewhere until the early hours. In 1916 he was contracted to form a trio with pianist José Martínez and bandoneonist Pedro Polito to play at a small venue at the 1916 carnival in Rosario. Whilst there he was asked to play in a city centre tearoom. In order to carry the music through the larger, fuller venue he had to call for reinforcements: Leopoldo Thompson arrived from Buenos Aires with his double bass and Rafael Rinaldi with his more portable violin. Canaro called this new quintet 'Pirincho' which was the nickname given to him at birth[129].

We have read above in the *Carnivals* section that Canaro joined forces with Roberto Firpo to provide a super-group, a grand orquesta típica, for the 1917 carnival in Rosario. Canaro was already a crowd-pleasing performer, a respected composer, an orchestra leader, and a popular recording artist but the Firpo-Canaro extravanganza was yet another boost to his accelerating career that would last until the 1960s. He made his last recordings on 29 July 1964, over 50 years after his first, and only five months before he passed away.

---

[129] his tuft of hair apparently resembled the head feathers of a pirincho bird

Juan D'Arienzo

On 14 December 1900 Juan D'Arienzo was born in central Buenos Aires to parents Alberto D'Arienzo and Amalia Améndola. Amalia encouraged her children to learn music and play the piano: Juan soon changed to the violin. His younger brother Ernani became a jazz pianist and drummer and his sister Josefina a pianist and singer. The 11-year-old Juan D'Arienzo, now a precocious violinist, was invited to play at the children's theatre in the Palermo Zoological Gardens and did so regularly on Sundays for almost a year alongside his child pianist friend Ángel D'Agostino. The two of them continued to cross paths. For example in 1915 both Juan and Ángel were playing together with the (much older 25-year-old) bandoneonist Juan Deambroggio providing the music at a silent cinema.

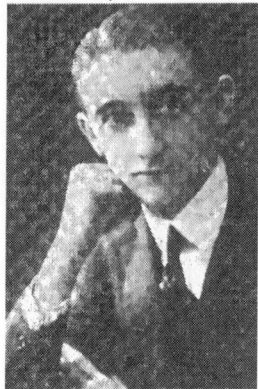

In 1918 D'Arienzo's uncle, Alfredo Améndola (the former owner of the Atlanta recording company [130]) introduced him to the famous tango composer, theatre producer and recording artist Arturo De Bassi[131]. Contacts (and in particular, family contacts) in the music business were always useful to help one's progress and D'Arienzo benefitted again 10 years later when Alfredo's son, Atilio Améndola, gave him his first break in to the recording studio at Electra Records. Meanwhile back in 1918 Arturo De Bassi employed Juan D'Arienzo as a violinist in a

---

[130] see *Recordings* above
[131] indirectly via Arturo's uncle Domingo De Bassi

musical production at the Teatro Avenida. A star of the show was the tango pioneer Carlos Posadas[132]. Nobody could have predicted the historic significance of their joint performance - the early pioneer and the later disrupter of tango dance music. It is surprising that, given this early boost to his career, D'Arienzo did not record any of Posada's compositions during the decades of his dance hall fame - waiting until near the end of his recording life in 1967 to record three of them *El jagüel*, *El tamango*, and *Cordón de oro*.

In late 1919 D'Arienzo was performing on the stage of the Teatro Nacional as a tango band in the play *El Cabaret Montmartre*. Alongside him was his long-time pianist friend Ángel D'Agostino, and his future friend and co-violinist Alfredo Mazzeo. Mazzeo served as first violinist on the D'Arienzo orchestra recordings from 1935 to 1939 and was responsible for producing the signature sound of the D'Arienzo dance orchestra - the low 'buzzing' of the bass string on the violin.

At the start of the 1920s D'Arienzo switched to playing jazz in the Select Jazz Band. There were no indications of the explosive impact he was to have in the world of tango a decade or so later.

Julio De Caro

José Guiseppe De Caro De Sica, had migrated from Italy (where he had held the position of Director of Music at the Teatro alla Scala in Milan) and was living in central Buenos Aires with his wife Mariana Ricciardi Villari. In March 1898 Mariana gave birth to a son, Francisco, and in December 1899 to Julio. The proud and

---

[132] who died that same year aged 43

ambitious father José not only tutored his children rigidly in European classical music in readiness for their pre-determined virtuoso careers but also dictated the specific instrument each would play. Up to 1907 Francisco had been learning the violin and Julio the piano but the children's first act of minor rebellion was to swap instruments (and in a further 10 years they would both abandon classical music for tango). Despite following their father's tuition and helping their father teach music to his students the brothers (still under 12 years old) were secretly playing the hit tangos by Bevilacqua, De Bassi, Greco and others, easily facilitated by the sheet music on sale in their father's music shop. They were further inspired by the tango musicians who visited the shop to browse and play the assorted instruments on display, Vicente Greco being amongst them.

In 1915 the adolescent Julio De Caro approached a friend of his father's, Cayetano De Bassi[133], who was directing a season of zarzuela plays at the city centre Teatro Lorea. Julio wanted to play violin in the theatre's orchestra. It was there that Julio got his taste of musical freedom, playing popular music for ordinary people rather than the controlled formal performances forced upon him by his father. When not in the orchestra pit Julio was visiting local cafés in order to hear the visiting tango musicians such as Roberto Firpo, Juan Carlos Cobián, and Eduardo Arolas. All this was without the knowledge of his father who was still clinging to more classical ambitions for his sons. In 1917 Julio went to see Firpo playing at the Palais De Glace in Recoleta and Julio's friends surprised him by forcing him up to the stage (vociferously encouraged by Eduardo Arolas who was also in the audience). The

---

[133] father of tango composer Arturo De Bassi

obliging Agesilao Ferrazzano[134] gave this unknown boy his violin and Julio played a well-known tango to much applause and appreciation by all, including the watching Arolas. Some weeks later Eduardo Arolas walked innocently in to the music shop of Don Guiseppe De Caro and told him how impressed he had been with Julio's tango performance. The revelation did not turn out well as Arolas was ushered out of the premises and Julio was forbidden to ever involve himself with tango again. Of course Julio was by now completely captivated by tango and did play in the Arolas quartet, as second violin to Rafael Tuegols. It was all too much for his father who banished Julio from his home and they become estranged for many years to come. The paternal aspirations of Don Guiseppe De Caro were further shattered when his other sons Francisco, Emilio, and José also chose the tango path.

At the end of 1917 in Café T.V.O, in the barrio of Barracas, Julio was temporarily standing in for the absent violinist of the Ricardo Brignolo orchestra. The pianist there was José María Rizzuti with whom Julio became great friends and musical companions. In the summer season of 1918 (December to February) De Caro and Rizutti travelled to Montevideo in the orchestra of Eduardo Arolas. A personal bonus for De Caro was that he was able to stay with his brother Francisco, who had escaped to Montevideo following his own break up with his father, and their time together resulted in several joint compositions of tangos. In February 1919 Julio De Caro and José Rizzuti left the Arolas orchestra and returned to Buenos Aires where they linked up with bandoneonist Pedro Maffia. They were performing in a local café when Osvaldo Fresedo entered to check out the pianist about whom he had heard many

---

[134] in his autobiography De Caro recalls incorrectly that it was 'Tito' Roccatagliata and that he played *La Cumparsita*

good reports. He offered Rizzuti a place in his new sextet. Rizutti accepted but only on the conditions that De Caro and Maffia were also accepted. The new Fresedo sextet with Rizzuti, De Caro, and Maffia started at the Casino Pigalle on 1 July 1919. The musicians were perfectly matched and the sextet became very popular very quickly however within a year it all changed when Fresedo abandoned his sextet and headed to New York.

Julio De Caro had learnt from the tango styles of Eduardo Arolas, Osvaldo Fresedo, and José María Rizutti and in the following decade would become a prolific composer and entrepreneurial orchestra leader leading to a era of elaborate tango music that has become known as 'Decarean' (that is, 'of De Caro').

Agesilao Ferrazzano

Born in 1897 in Buenos Aires, Agesilao Ferrazzano trained as a violinist and came to the attention of the tango scene in 1914. The pianist Roberto Firpo had invited him as second violinist to

support his lead violin David 'Tito' Roccatagliata, alongside bandoneonist Juan Deambroggio, and flautist Alejando Michetti. Ferrazzano demonstrated such skilful creativity in melancholic and lyrical counter-melodies to Tito's pizzicato and rhythmic lead that, together with Firpo's innovative compositions, the new quintet produced a level of sophistication hitherto unheard in a tango orchestra. Ferrazzano at the age of 17 had established himself as a talented tango violinist and master of the

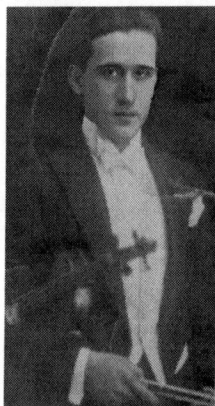

violin *contracanto* (a soon-to-be obligatory sound of orquestas típicas). He was still with Firpo in 1917 and therefore part of the super-sized orchestra of Firpo-Canaro in Rosario. As Roccatagliata had recently left the orchestra Ferrazzano was promoted to first violin and the new recruit to the second violin position was 15-year-old Cayetano Puglisi. Late in 1918 Ferrazzano also left Firpo and joined the quintet of bandoneonist Juan Guido before teaming up with pianist Vicente Gorrese to create a quintet suitably named Gorrese-Ferrazzano. That venture was short-lived but the two got together later as part of the new Orquesta Típica Victor from 1925 to 1931.

Ferrazzano spent the 1920s playing in the top tier of tango orchestras before deciding to travel to Europe.

Cayetano Puglisi

In 1909 Cayetano Puglisi, aged 7, arrived with his family in Buenos Aires from Italy and by 1914 was playing violin alongside the bandoneonist Carlos Marcucci in the Trio de Pibes (the Three Kids) at the Bar Iglesias in the centre of the city on Calle Corrientes.

At the age of 15 he joined the quintet of Roberto Firpo as second violinist to Agesilao Ferrazzano. His new colleagues taught him the general tango sound that they required and specifically the playful counter-melodies. Being in such a high-profile band Puglisi had to meet the audience's expectations from the start and he certainly did not disappoint. When Ferrazzano left the orchestra in 1918 Cayetano Puglisi stepped up to the position of first violin and Roberto Firpo rewarded him with the name of his latest tango composition *El talento*. On the cover of the printed sheet music is Firpo's personal dedication 'To my respected companion C. Puglisi the youngest and most eminent tango violinist - my admiration'. Praise indeed.

Cayetano Puglisi could have had no better musical home than Roberto Firpo's orchestra and so he stayed for the next decade during which time Firpo's admiration for him did not diminish.

David 'Tito' Roccatagliata

David Roccatagliata was born in 1891 in Buenos Aires and, thanks to a formal education in classical music, became an outstanding violinist. His introduction to a professional tango career came in 1908 when pianist Roberto Firpo and clarinetist Juan Carlos Bazán expanded their duo to a trio At some point during his adolescence he picked up the nickname of 'Tito' that stayed with him for the rest of his (short) life. In 1909 he joined the quartet of Eduardo Arolas. Both of them were 18 years old, playing the late night bars and living what in much later times was described as the rock and roll lifestyle. There was nothing inevitable about Tito's dissolute life but it came to define him and remained a strong undercurrent beneath all of his glorious musical creativity. Over the next decade both Arolas and Roccatagliata became addicted to alcohol and drugs and both were dead before they reached their mid-thirties.

Roccatagliata played alongside other great tango pioneers such as bandoneonist Arturo Bernstein in 1910. In 1912 he was at the Café Argentino playing in a quartet with bandoneonist Graciano De Leone, pianist Agustin Bardi and flautist Carlos Hernani Macchi.

His style was similar to that of Ernesto Ponzio, peppered with lots of playful pizzicato plucking. He was recruited by Genaro Espósito to form a trio with Roberto Firpo and they played at the top venues such as the Armenonville and Café Estribo. They recorded 10 tangos on the Columbia label as the Orquesta Típica Gennaro. In their publicity Tito Roccatagliata was described as the famous criollo violinist. In 1914 the trio auditioned to become the house band for the Armenonville but the management selected only Roberto Firpo. Firpo took Roccatagliata with him and replaced Espósito with Eduardo Arolas. Once again the party-loving Roccatagliata and Arolas were back together. Later that year Firpo recruited a second violinist, the 17-year-old Agesilao Ferrazzano, who provided the lyrical counter-melodies to Roccatagliata's rhythmic pizzicato style.

He remained a constant in Firpo's quintet until early 1917. The reasons for his departure are unknown but what happened afterwards may shed some light. Almost immediately after his departure he joined bandoneonist Manuel Pizarro to form a quartet and in May 1917 they went on a tour of the province of La Pampa. Pizarro recalled that their agent cancelled their engagements after only three days due to Roccatagliata's constant drunkenness and his harassment of the hotel's cleaning maids. That should have come as no surprise to Pizarro because several years earlier he had previously toured with Roccatagliata and Ernesto Ponzio and remembered them both as being drunken, disorderly and, in Ponzio's case, quite violent.

It is a testament to Roccatagliata's creative genius that, despite all of the obvious personal flaws, the professional musicians continued to seek him out. Still in 1917 he was once again with Eduardo Arolas playing with pianist Juan Carlos Cobían. Arolas composed a 'tango sentimental' that he named *Lágrimas* (Tears) that is best known today by the 1941 version by Ricardo Tanturi. Arolas dedicated it to the mother of his friend David 'Tito' Roccatagliata and the illustration on the front of the sheet music is heartbreaking. It shows a mother in tears whilst arriving at the door is the drunken son holding a bottle of alcohol and a violin case.

Arolas soon left to pursue other musical adventures and was replaced by the 20-year-old Osvaldo Fresedo. Despite Roccatgliata's obvious problems with alcohol he, Cobían, and Fresedo thrived as friends and as innovative musicians. When Fresedo was offered a contract in 1920 to record in the USA Victor studios as the Orquesta Típica Select he took with him his friend and tango genius Roccatagliata. Sadly, but predictably, his weaknesses remained. Rocccatagliata died in 1925 and left us only four compositions, the most familiar to us today is *Elegante papirusa* recorded by Edgardo Donato (1935).

6.   Flautists

Macchi, Pecci, Michetti, Pugliese

<u>Carlos Macchi</u>

Carlos Hernani Macchi was born in 1878 and became a respected contributor to, and influencer of, the emerging tango sound and often the musical brain behind those pioneers whose names are now more familiar than his. He grew up in a family home of instruments and it was his older brother that taught him how to play the violin. By the 1890s he was playing polkas, mazurkas, milongas, and tangos in duets and trios in the streets and café-bars around the busy Abasto market. By 1907 he had played with the guitarist Eusebio Aspiazú and the flautist Luis Teisseire and shortly afterwards, perhaps inspired by Teisseire, he put his violin to one side and became a tango flautist putting him at the core of tango groups and recordings for the next decade.

In the first couple of years of the 1910s he was playing with bandoneonists Graciano De Leone and separately with Juan Maglio with whom he recorded his own compositions: *El reservado* and *Sarita*. In 1910 he performed in a quartet at the café La Morocha on the Calle Corrientes with bandoneonist Domingo Santa Cruz, Domingo's brother Juan Santa Cruz, and violinist Julio Orioli (who was later later replaced by Alcides Palavecino). The photograph below (published on 29 April 1913 in the magazine Sherlock Holmes) shows Macchi seated on the right with his flute upon his lap, behind him is violinist Alcides Palavecino, at the piano is Juan Santa Cruz, and seated with his bandoneón is Domingo Santa Cruz. Domingo composed and dedicated the tango *Hernani* to Macchi who reciprocally composed the tango *Santa Cruz* dedicating it to the brothers Domingo and Juan and describing it on his sheet music as a 'tango cariñoso' (tango with affection). Unfortunately neither of those tangos are heard today as they were not amongst the limited discography of the relatively few orchestras that fill today's tango dance floors.

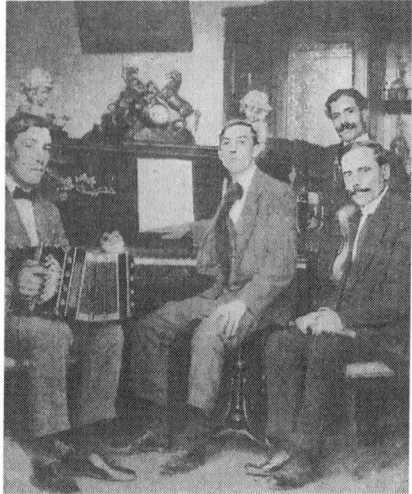

Macchi formed and directed the Cuarteto Típica Criollo La Armonia with José 'Pepino' Bonano (violin), Juan Manuel Firpo (bandoneón), and Leopoldo Thompson (guitar). In 1914 the quartet made several recordings including *El jaguel* and *El apache argentino* that are tangos still heard today thanks to the recordings of later orchestras (Carlos Di Sarli and Aníbal Troilo). They also recorded Macchi's own composition, *Pepino*, dedicated to his violinist. You can listen to that original *Pepino* recording on YouTube. Unusually the record label named each of the musicians and their instruments although Firpo's is described as a 'Bandoleón' which was not an unusual spelling at that time.

In July 1916, in New York, the Victor Orchestra recorded Macchi's tango composition *Sarita* for a wider, non-tango-orientated, audience. The North American musicians played piano, four violins, flute, bass clarinet, cornet, viola, cello, bassoon, and a trombone, but not a bandoneón. In 1917 Macchi was back in the Juan Maglio quartet, again alongside José 'Pepino' Bonano, and in April recorded over 20 tracks on the Victor label.

Carlos Hernani Macchi was more than a flautist. He was able to play (and teach others to play) the violin, piano, and bandoneón. He could read and write musical notation. He understood the theory of music and how to arrange several instruments. He assisted Juan Maglio, Eduardo Arolas, and Agustín Bardi (amongst many others) to improve their arrangements and he transcribed their compositions so that they could publish them and earn a few pesos. He composed many tangos himself, although unfortunately none were subsequently recorded by the later orchestras and so have not reached the ears of today's tango fans.

Vicente Pecci

Vicente Pecci was born in Italy in 1886 and by the age of 13 he was in Buenos Aires playing the flute. In 1900 he was playing tangos with pianist Enrique Saborido and violinist Ernesto Ponzio. From 1910 to 1919 he was the favourite choice of the ground-breaking orquestas típicas of Vicente Greco, Genaro Espósito, and Eduardo Arolas and we can hear Pecci on their recordings during those years. Pecci was great friends with all of the emerging tango stars, and the closest and most long-standing of all was Ernesto Ponzio.

Pecci brought up his son, Juan, in to the world of tango and had asked Ernesto Ponzio to be Juan's godfather. In 1916 Ponzio was teaching Juan Pecci not only how to play violin but how to play it with swing and lots of pizzicato playfulness, namely in the Ponzio-style. Juan Pecci recalled that when he played a piece particularly well his teacher and godfather Ponzio, rather than being pleased, quickly become jealous and dismissive. Vicente Pecci took his son Juan to his tango gigs and introduced him to the big names like Domingo Santa Cruz, Juan Maglio and Eduardo Arolas. The pioneer tango flautist saw his son enter the new wave of tango orchestras. Peccci Junior was soon playing alongside the adolescent Juan D'Arienzo and in about 1922 went to Paris to join Eduardo Bianco, staying in Europe until the 1950s.

In 1920 Vicente Pecci diversified in to theatre productions and wrote the music for the play *Las Golondrinas* which, unsurprisingly, incorporated tango music and dance. Pecci continued playing through the 1920s but was by then outside of the mainstream tango orchestras. He represented the earlier era of tango and so for him a perfect opportunity came along at the start of the 1930s when he was invited by his good friend Ernesto Ponzio to join the revival group of the Orquesta Típica de la Guardia Vieja. He was to play alongside his other pioneer friends Enrique Saborido and Eusebio Aspiazü. In 1942, at the Teatro Apolo, at the age of 56 he appeared in a production based on the evolution of tango from Villoldo to Gardel[135] where he played the historically important character of...Vicente Pecci.

---

[135] *La Cabalgata del Tango, de Villoldo a Gardel*

Alejandro Michetti

Alejandro Michetti was born in Italy in 1896 and came to Argentina with his parents in 1899. At the age of ten he started to play the flute professionally in the silent cinemas. At 16 he joined the tango orchestra of Roberto Firpo and within a year Firpo recorded Michetti's tango composition *Quién te iguala,* which is better known today by the recording of Carlos Di Sarli (1952). Michetti stayed with Firpo and was therefore on many of his recordings until 1927 (with a short break in 1917 whilst he was touring with the other tango giant Juan Maglio). He also briefly formed and recorded as his own orquesta criolla. Michetti never came to terms with the loss of the flute from the tango orchestras and said that the replacement bandoneón could never adequately match the beautiful tones of the flute. We can admire his dedication to his beloved instrument but it was not an emotional attachment shared by the majority of tango enthusiasts at that time.

Adolfo Pugliese

Adolfo Pugliese was a leather worker during the day but his passion was music and his idea of relaxation after a full day's work was to join his friends at local café-bars in the barrio of Villa Crespo and play tangos on his flute. His other passion was Aurelia who he had married in 1898 and the following year had a son Vicente, followed two years later by Alberto, and in 1905 by a third son Osvaldo. Adolfo Pugliese was keen that his sons should also become musicians and over the next few years he encouraged them all to learn the violin. It did not take long for him to realise that having three young boys at home all scratching various sounds out of the violin did not make the most harmonious domestic scene nor create a potential home tango group. So for some variety he decided to steer his youngest, Osvaldo, towards piano lessons but was met with considerable resistance. His son was not the most diligent of students, neither at school nor at home. Adolfo persisted and one day when Osvaldo returned home from his work at a printing company Adolfo presented his son with a present – his own piano and the name of an outstanding teacher. Adolfo took Osvaldo with him to his tango gigs to experience the music and the appreciation of the café customers. When Osvaldo became more proficient on the piano, and there was a piano at the venue, Adolfo encouraged his son to join the group and get some practice in front of dancers.

Adolfo Pugliese is an example of one of the many tango musicians in the early 1900s that opened the pathways for the generation that went on to create the recorded music danced at 21st century milongas around the world. From the mid-1920s Adolfo's son, Osvaldo Pugliese, went on to join some of the best tango groups and in the 1940s directed his own orchestra and made recordings until 1986. Osvaldo Pugliese remains a clear favourite of tango fans today, whether dancers or not.

7.   Guitarists

Camarano, Thompson

Félix Camarano

In 1908 the guitarist Félix Camarano was playing the café-bars in La Boca and in particular at La Marina with, then violinist, Agustín Bardi. Also in that year he played in a quartet with the guitarist-turned-bandoneonist Arturo Severino. Guitars were slowly going out of favour amongst tango musicians as the genre was being defined by the bandoneón, piano, violin, and double bass. The guitarists Graciano de Leone and Ricardo González both switched to bandoneón; guitarists Samuel Castriota and Luciano Ríos to piano; and guitarists Leopoldo Thompson and Rodolfo Duclós to double bass. Félix Camarano, on the other hand, did not abandon his guitar and tango fans did not abandon him.

In 1912 Camarano was in a quartet led by bandoneonist Genaro Espósito and on two days in January and February recorded some 20 tracks on the Victor label[136]. By 1916 he was directing his own tango orquesta típica, still as a guitarist, and was contracted by Carlos Nasca (of the ERA record company) to make a series of recordings. Understandably he chose some of the most popular compositions of the day which remain equally popular today:

---

[136] see *Bandoneonists/Espósito* above

TITLE	BEST KNOWN RECORDED VERSIONS
Charamusca	Francisco Canaro (1934, 1950), Juan D'Arienzo (1939);
Pollito	Francisco Canaro (1927, 1931), Juan D'Arienzo (1938), Carlos Di Sarli (1947, 1951)
El flete	Francisco Canaro (1928, 1939), Juan D'Arienzo (1936)
Germaine	Carlos Di Sarli (1941, 1951, 1955)
Entre dos fuegos	Juan D'Arienzo (1940)
Lágrimas	Roberto Firpo (1940), Ricardo Tanturi (1941), Juan D'Arienzo (1947)
La rosarina	Orquesta Típica Victor (1929), Roberto Firpo (1936), Juan D'Arienzo (1937), Francisco Canaro (1943).

As ever, when we listen to tango recordings by our favourite orchestras from the 1930s all the way to the modern day we are frequently listening to a tango story that is more, often much more, than a century old.

Leopoldo Thompson

By this period Leopoldo Thompson was a long established masterful guitarist who also provided percussion by slapping the strings and the wooden guitar body and using a nine-string guitar[137] to provide a powerful bass. In 1911 he was performing with the popular violinist Ernesto Ponzio and the rising star bandoneonist Eduardo Arolas. By 1913 he was the guitarist in the quartet of pianist Roberto Firpo at the high-class cabaret Armenonville and at the café El Estribo with Eduardo Arolas (bandoneón) and David 'Tito' Roccatagliata (violin). That same year he replaced the guitarist Luciano Ríos in the quartet of Juan Maglio.

In 1916 he upgraded his instrument to a double bass and played in the Quinteto Pirincho at the Rosario carnival with violinist Francisco Canaro, pianist José Martínez, Pedro Polito on bandoneón, and second violinist Rafael Rinaldi. It was his contribution to that quintet that elevated the double bass to become a standard instrument in the orquesta típica line-up although nobody played it quite like Thompson. He continued his energetic style of guitar-playing (by using the palm of his hand to slap, and his fingers to drum upon, the strings and the wooden body of his instrument) but with the double bass he also had the arc of the bow to bounce on the strings like a

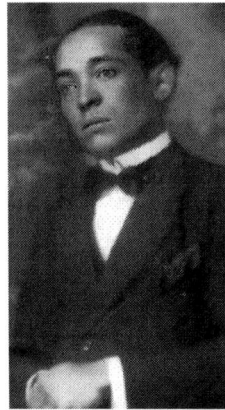

---

[137] guitars varied and had from 6 to 10 strings to provide the necessary depth of bass

drum beat. Holding his left hand across the neck of the double bass, deadening the vibration, he scraped his bow across the strings for an extra earthy effect. As if that was not enough to drive the audience wild his added speciality was to call out and add vocal sound effects to keep everyone, his fellow musicians included, pumped up and then in his most excitable moments he danced around and around the double bass, whilst still playing.

He went on to play for the more sedate and sophisticated sextets of Osvaldo Fresedo and Julio De Caro but in 1925 he suffered a short illness and died suddenly, aged only 35.

The Continuing Story

The story of tango and its pioneers continues in the series *Get To Know the Tango Pioneers* with linked on-line music tracks and film clips:

Myths and the Melting Pot: Origins to 1909

There was a vibrant tango scene in live performances and recordings in the years up to 1909. A fertile environment was developing in which future tango stars were growing up and absorbing the culture around them. We see the emergence of Ángel Villoldo, Arturo De Bassi, Enrique Saborido, Eduardo Arolas, Vicente Greco, Juan Maglio, Francisco Canaro and many others.

The Precarious Years: 1920 to 1935

Despite the threat of imported jazz we see the growth of tango in recordings, the theatre, films with sound, and the new technological reach of radio. We also see the emergence of poets and singers, and of musicians and orchestra leaders that are familiar to today's tango fans, including: Rodolfo Biagi, Miguel Caló, Lucio Demare, Edgardo Donato, Pedro Laurenz, Osvaldo Pugliese, Ricardo Tanturi, and Aníbal Troilo.

Arrabal: technically the outer edges of the city but in general usage indicating the lower-class areas and people, regardless of geography
Bandoneón: a musical instrument, like a concertina, with buttons rather than piano keys and is almost exclusively associated with tango
Barrio: an area in a city, often with a distinct characteristic
Candombe: a drum-based rhythm associated with African origin
Compadrito: a young man who is, or is trying to appear, cool
Conventillo: over-crowded social housing with a shared patio space
Criollo: creole, of mixed ethnic origin
Gaucho: a non-city dweller elevated by literature to an heroic figure
Habanera: music and dance style named after Havana (Cuba) also known as 'tango americano'
Milonga: a national song; a post-1932 dance rhythm; a dance event
Organito: a portable mechanical instrument with bellows
Orquesta Típica: a group of musicians playing tango dance music, with bandoneón
Payador: a singer/guitarist of melancholic, traditionally improvised, verse
Porteño: a resident of Buenos Aires
Quebrada: a dance move associated with, but preceded, tango
Rondalla: a group of musicians playing stringed instruments
Tango andaluz: from Southern Spain also called Tango Gitano (Gypsy) and Tango Flamenco
Tango argentino: I use this to denote the musical genre that emerged from Buenos Aires in the early 1900s
Tango canción: a sung tango, not for the dance market
Vals: an alternative spelling of waltz
Zarzuela: a Spanish theatre play with song and dance, the sainete is a variant as is the revista but is (generally) without music.

Images

The illustrations and photographs have been reproduced with the kind permission of:

Archivo General de la Nación de Argentina, Buenos Aires, Argentina;

Biblioteca Nacional de España, Madrid, Spain;

Ibero-Amerikanisches Institut, Berlin, Germany;

the Ferrazzano family (page 198);

the Medrano family for the illustration *La Cumparsita* (page 6);

author photograph (p222) and cover artwork courtesy of Adrian Cubitt;

other images are sourced from material in the Public Domain.

Cover illustration published in Buenos Aires 1909.

On-line material includes the complete collection at the:
- Biblioteca Nacional de España, (Hemeroteca Digital);
- Ibero-Amerikanisches Institut;
- Discography of American Historical Recordings;
- UCSB Cylinder Audio Archive;
- Library of Congress; and the
- Archivo General de la Nación de Argentina.

A multitude of other websites have provided access to newspapers, magazines, photographs, record labels, discographies, recordings, population census, genealogy, travel and migration information.

Published works include:
- A city of trades: Spanish and Italian Immigrants in Late 19th Century Buenos Aires (for the European Historical Economics Society) *Blanca Sánchez-Alonso*
- Argentina 1516-1987 *David Rock*
- Between the Gaucho and the Tango...1895–1915 *Brian Bockelman*
- Blackness and Urban Popular Sectors in Buenos Aires (1895-1916) *Lea Geler*
- Buenos Aires: Arrabal-Sainete-Tango, *Domingo Casadevall*
- Buenos Aires Setenta Años Atrás *Dr. José Antonio Wilde*
- Carlos Gardel *Simon Collier*
- Cine Argentino *Octavio Getin,*
- Cosas de negros *Vicente Rossi*
- Doce Ventanas del Tango *Fundación El Libro*
- El Arte del Payador *Raúl Dorra*
- El Encanto de Buenos Aires *Gómez Carillo*
- El tango argentino como espejo de la sociedad en su

Bibliography

contexto histórico *Professor Dr. Christian Wentzlaff-Eggebert*

- El Tango Argentino de Salon *Nicanor Lima*
- El Tango en la sociedad porteña 1880-1920 *Hugo Lamas & Enrique Binda*
- El Tango en Mis Recuerdos *Julio De Caro*
- El Tango su Historia y Evolución *Horacio Ferrer*
- En Argentine de Buenos Aires au Gran Chaco *Jules Huret*
- Entre Cortes y Quebradas, Candombes, Milongas, y Tangos en su Historia y Comentarios *Pintín Castellanos*
- Entre fonógrafos y radios: difusión del tango durante las primeras décadas del siglo XX *Andrea Matallana*
- Evarista Carriego *Jorge Luis Borges*
- Fábricas de Músicas *Marina Cañardo*
- Folklore en el Uruguay, La Guitarra del Gaucho, Sus Danzas y Canciones *Cedar Viglietti*
- Herencia Africana en el Tango 1870-1890 *Gustavo Goldman*
- Immigrants in the Lands of Promise: Italians in Buenos Aires and New York. *Samuel L. Baily*
- La Historia de la Orquesta Típica *Luis Adolfo Sierra*
- La Historia del Tango Volumes 1 to 18 *published by Corregidor*
- La música en los inicios del cine sonoro argentino *Rosa Chalkho*
- Las Raices del Tango *Eduardo Giorlandini*
- Lo Criollo en el Tango *Susana Ibarburu*
- Los Primeros 25 Años de la Fonográfia Argentina *Enrique Binda*
- Mis Memorias *Francisco Canaro*
- Music Trade Review magazines 1905 - 1928
- Nueva Historia del Tango *Héctor Benedetti*
- Otros tangos origenes mediaticos del tango en el teatro y

215

la danza *Jimena Anabel Jauregui,*

- Popular, Elite and Mass Culture The Spanish Zarzuela in Buenos Aires 1890-1900 *Kristen McCleary*
- Recording Studios on Tour: The Expeditions of the Victor Talking Machine Company through Latin America 1903-1926, a dissertation by *Sergio Daniel Ospina Romero*
- Sainete y cine sonoro argentino *Alicia Aisemberg*
- Talking Machine Review magazines 1905-1927
- Tango Testigo Social *Andrés Carretero*
- Tango Aborigen *Marisa Uthurralt & Alberto González Arzac*
- The Afro-Argentines of Buenos Aires 1800-1900 *George Reid Andrews*
- The Argentina Reader *published by Gabriela Nouzeilles & Graciela Montaldo*
- The Art History of Love *Robert Farris Thompson*
- The Invention of Argentina *Nicolas Shunway*
- The Quest for the Embrace *Gustavo Benzecry Sabá*
- The Zonophone Record 1901-1903 *Ernie Bayly & Michael Kinnear*

Additionally I have researched several hundred book extracts, academic papers, opinion pieces, articles, interviews, letters, and collations of multiple sources and so I apologise for the inevitable omission from the above list of other contributing information.

The Author

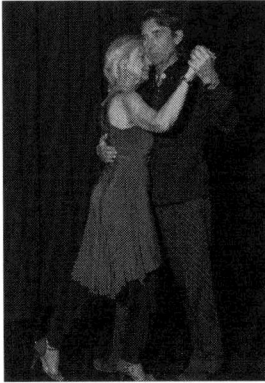

David's research in to the history of Argentine tango precedes the authorship of this book by over a decade, and continues today.

His investigative methods draw on his professional background: for over 30 years David served in several UK national intelligence and investigation agencies. He much prefers applying his skills (securing multiple corroborative sources to identify people, their associates, and their activities) to the more cultural world of tango.

In 2021/2022 David completed a Diploma course (*La Historia del Tango*) with the Instituto Argentino del Tango, Buenos Aires, Argentina.

David presents seminars on *Get To Know the Tango Orchestras* and *Get To Know the Tango Pioneers*. He enjoys dancing tango, is a tango DJ and (with his wife Marion) organises milongas and tango classes. At time of publication he is also Chairman of the UK Argentine Tango Association.